the
BELLY
FAT *Diet*
COOKBOOK

105 Easy and Delicious Recipes to Lose Your Belly, Shed Excess Weight, Improve Health

JOHN CHATHAM

CONTENTS

INTRODUCTION

Everything we think we know about belly fat is wrong. Until recently, nutrition and health experts had fairly firm beliefs about how to lose belly fat. One had to stick to a low-calorie, low-fat diet and spend a lot of time in the gym on strenuous cardio exercises and abdominal workouts. However, recent research into how and why our bodies store and use belly fat has led to revolutionary new thinking about transforming our bodies into lean, toned, fat-burning machines. And guess what? You don't have to live the life of an athlete or eat like a bird to lose that belly fat. In fact, by following the Belly Fat Diet plan and eating healthfully, you'll get dramatic results faster than you ever thought possible, and you'll do it without being miserable or sacrificing your health.

Chapter One of this book explains the dangers of excess belly fat, the myths we have about losing belly fat, what you can expect from the diet, and how the diet works. Chapter Two gets you ready to choose the right foods and avoid the ones that will make losing belly fat more difficult. Chapter Three gives you some lists of smart food choices while shopping so you're ready for Chapters Four through Thirteen, which will give you the recipes for success—more than one hundred delicious, easy-to-prepare meals for every part of your day. Recipes that you can enjoy without the guilt usually associated with diets.

Losing stubborn belly fat isn't about calorie counting, avoiding all fats, and countless abdominal crunches—in fact, you can toss all these aside. A flat stomach is actually faster, easier, and more pleasant than anything you could have imagined, and your only difficulty with the Belly Fat Diet and the recipes in this book will be remembering that you're on a diet at all.

THE BASICS OF THE BELLY FAT DIET

According to renowned cardiologist and author Dr. Mehmet Oz, one's waist measurement is the most important indicator of overall health. If your waist measurement is more than half your height (in inches), according to Dr. Oz, you are at serious risk for heart disease, stroke, and type 2 diabetes. This statement has caused many people to look at their measuring tapes not just as a way to measure their fitness but also as a way to measure their future.

The Dangers of Excess Belly Fat

Belly Fat Damages Your Liver

Several recent studies on the connection between obesity (particularly excess belly fat) and high levels of liver fat have shown that there is a much higher rate of fatty liver in those with excess belly fat. Fatty liver is a leading indicator of several lipid and metabolic disorders and even liver cancer. In these studies, researchers found that liver fat is strongly associated with increased secretion of very low-density lipoproteins (VLDL), which contain the highest amount of triglycerides. High levels of triglycerides carry an increased risk of metabolic abnormalities, heart disease, and premature death.

Belly Fat Increases Insulin Resistance and Type 2 Diabetes

When we eat, our food, especially carbohydrates, is broken down into glucose so that it can be used to power every cell in our bodies. However, to be used as energy rather than stored as fat, glucose requires the help of insulin, a hormone secreted by the pancreas.

Insulin's job is to serve as a key that unlocks your body's cells so that glucose can enter and be used by the cells as energy. Fat cells, particularly abdominal fat cells, lessen the sensitivity to insulin, making it harder for glucose to pass through cell walls. Because the glucose can't enter the cells, it remains in the bloodstream (high blood sugar). The pancreas responds by producing and releasing more insulin. This cycle repeats itself and grows worse over time. This is what leads to metabolic syndrome and type 2 diabetes.

Belly Fat Increases the Risk of Heart Disease and Stroke

Because belly fat is so close to the liver (and often accompanied by excess fat directly surrounding the liver), it boosts production of LDL cholesterol (the one we don't want boosted!). This cholesterol eventually becomes a waxy substance known as plaque, which sticks to artery walls and eventually causes swelling, narrowing the arteries. This narrowing increases blood pressure, which seriously taxes the heart. It also increases your chance of blood clots, which can cause stroke.

Belly Fat Increases the Risk of Dementia

Excess belly fat has even been linked to an increased risk of dementia. In fact, excess belly fat increases your risk of developing dementia by as much as 145 percent! This is a result of the same inflammation in the artery walls, which decreases proper blood flow to the brain.

With all of the serious health risks linked to belly fat, it's easy to see that getting rid of excess belly fat should be a very high priority. Fortunately, while we have lots of scary research that shows the risks of belly fat, we also have all of the new research that shows us how to get rid of belly fat quickly, easily, and permanently.

Belly Fat Myths

Myth #1: Excess Belly Fat Is Your Destiny

Fact: This long-held belief about losing belly fat has led to a great deal of frustration for dieters. Research studies have found that it has been our approach to dieting that has caused people to give up—not heredity.

Myth #2: Low-Calorie Diets Decrease Belly Fat

Fact: For decades, it was accepted that the only way to lose fat was to take in fewer calories than you use. There are a few things that make this difficult. First, cutting calories does not specifically address losing belly fat. Second, counting calories leads to people eating too few calories. Since this is difficult to maintain, it often leads to yo-yo dieting cycles as well as reaching the infamous "weight-loss plateau," where your metabolism adjusts to the lowered caloric intake and virtually shuts down.

Myth #3: Dietary Fat Is the Enemy

Fact: All fat is not bad. In fact, fat is an essential nutrient. Fat not only enhances the flavor of food, it also gives us a feeling of satisfaction and fullness. It is also used to transport essential vitamins and minerals. The key is not to cut out all fat but to cut out the bad trans-fats and cut down on saturated fats, which are found primarily in animal products such as meat and butter. Healthy fats improve our heart health and brain function, and help us lose belly fat.

Myth #4: Burning Tons of Calories Is the Answer

The other long-held belief about losing belly fat was that you had to burn it off by spending hours at the gym. This approach did not specifically target the loss of belly fat. Many people spent hours on the treadmill or in aerobics classes and saw the numbers on the scale drop while the belly fat stayed put. This is why we saw a surge in popular diets that claimed to work with your "set point" of weight or BMI, or to address certain body types.

Thankfully, we now know that these methods and theories simply failed to address the ways and the reasons that our bodies are designed to store fat or dispose of belly fat. While our genetics and heredity may decide whether we have a long torso or wide shoulders, whether we tend to store fat on our hips or on our thighs, they do not mean that some people can have flat abs and some can't.

Myth #5: Abdominal Crunches Helps Lose Belly Fat

For years, it was accepted as fact that in order to lose belly fat, you had to do specific exercises that targeted the abs. People spent hours doing sit-ups or crunches without seeing results. There's a very simple reason for this: resistance exercise does not burn fat in a specific area. Exercise burns calories and speeds up your metabolism, but your body doesn't burn fat from your abs because you're doing crunches. Resistance exercises such as crunches build and tone lean abdominal muscles, but your muscles are located beneath (or behind) the fat layer. In order for those crunches to result in a flat, toned tummy, you have to get rid of the fat that's hiding those muscles.

What You Can Expect From the Belly Fat Diet

You Will Lose Weight

Because most diets are designed to help you lose weight by cutting and/ or burning calories, they result in weight loss that includes the loss of stored water and lean muscle tissue. If you're able to stick to them for long, you may see a nice new number on the scale, but you still look flabby because you've lost muscle instead of stored fat.

This plan does not rely on simply cutting calories to lose weight. The key is that you will be taking in the right calories—from foods that actually help to speed up your metabolism, burn stored fat, and utilize your food better to provide energy.

You Will Not Be Counting Calories, Carbs, or Fat Grams

The Foods List in Chapter Two is designed to provide plenty of nutrition and satisfaction without empty calories, excess carbs, or unhealthful fats. As long as you stick to the Foods List and follow some simple guidelines, there's no need to track everything you put in your mouth.

You Will Not Be Portioning or Weighing Anything

One of the reasons that most diets fail, even diets that are based on solid science, is that they take too much time to follow correctly. No matter how good a diet is, if you don't have time to follow it, it won't work for you. By sticking to the Foods List and following some simple guidelines, you will get plenty of food and nutrients without getting too much fat or too many unhealthy carbs.

You Will Not Be Hungry All the Time

One of the keys to losing belly fat is to eat as frequently as possible, even grazing all day long. Because of this, you won't have to be left feeling hungry or have to suffer through cravings brought on by too little food or a lack of the right nutrients.

You Will Not Be Tired and Grumpy

Frequent meals and snacks keep your blood sugar steady. Spikes in blood sugar are quickly followed by crashes in blood sugar, leaving you feeling fatigued, foggy, and irritable. This is the cycle that occurs when you skip meals and then eat a large meal, or get too hungry and grab a snack filled with sugar. The Belly Fat Diet allows you to eat whenever you want—but you're also eating a diet rich in healthful carbs and fats, so you have a steady supply of energy without all those spikes and crashes.

You Will Lose Weight Faster than You Expect

It used to be accepted as fact that you should never lose more than two pounds per week. This is because most diets cut calories to lose weight. Losing more than two pounds per week meant that you were reducing your caloric intake to unhealthful levels and your body was feeding on its own muscle tissue as a source of protein and energy. Because the Belly Fat Diet does not rely on this method, but rather helps your body to reset and maximize its fat-burning and fat-storing systems, you can safely lose more than two pounds per week. The weight you lose will be stored fat, not lean muscle.

The Top Five Tools for Losing Belly Fat

The Belly Fat Diet takes all of the current research and all of the new findings about losing belly fat and incorporates them into one effective and easy-to-follow plan.

Tool #1: Breaking the Cortisol Cycle

Cortisol is one of the stress hormones naturally produced and secreted in the body. Cortisol's specific job is to react to stress signals by storing fat in the abdominal area. The reason this system exists is because, in ages past, stress often indicated a chance of famine in the near future. Back when people moved from place to place to find food and were often considered food themselves by other predators, stress was a signal that we were on the run and food was going to be in short supply.

Very few of us are in danger of famine from the stress we're under today, but we're more stressed today than people have ever been before. And this stress triggers the release of cortisol, which causes our bodies to direct fat to the abdomen to be used in case of famine. The problem is, there is no famine. We continue to eat more than enough food, so that fat is never used as an energy source.

The Belly Fat Diet will break the cortisol cycle and reset your system so that your body uses dietary fat properly and also gets rid of the fat it already has stored on your abdomen.

Tool #2: Reversing Insulin Resistance

Like cortisol, insulin is a hormone produced by your body, although it is not a stress hormone. The role of insulin is to regulate the amount of sugar in your bloodstream and to allow glucose (created from the foods you eat) to be used by cells as energy. You may have heard about insulin resistance, which is a situation where your body's cells become resistant to insulin and glucose cannot pass through the cell membrane to be used as energy. When this occurs, two things happen:

- Your blood sugar levels spike and drop repeatedly, causing a fatigue–energy boost–fatigue cycle.

- All of that unused glucose is stored as fat, mainly around your belly.

Like the situation with stress, cortisol, and belly fat, insulin resistance is cyclical. The cycle goes something like this:

- Excess belly fat makes your body resistant to insulin.

- Insulin resistance causes your body to store more belly fat.

This cycle is what can eventually lead to type 2 diabetes, which is why excess belly fat is a leading indicator of developing the disease. Fortunately, this cycle is reversible. In fact, even if you already have type 2 diabetes, losing belly fat and making the dietary changes prescribed in the Belly Fat Diet can greatly improve and even reverse the disease!

Tool #3: Vitamin C

Vitamin C has always been known as the wonder vitamin when it comes to preventing and relieving colds and other infections. However, the importance of vitamin C goes far beyond fighting infection and boosting immunity. It is also one of the key players in losing belly fat. It does this in two ways:

- First, vitamin C is a necessary for the production of L-carnitine, a chemical used to transport stored fat, particularly abdominal fat, to where it can be burned as energy.

- Second, vitamin C reduces the effects of stress on the body, which helps to break the cortisol cycle, so that your body is stimulated to both burn stored belly fat and to stop storing new belly fat.

On the Belly Fat Diet plan, you'll be getting a great deal of vitamin C from your diet, which will be full of vitamin C–dense foods. But you'll also be taking a vitamin C supplement twice per day to give your body the extra C it needs to burn the belly fat you already have.

Tool #4: Getting Leptin and Ghrelin on Your Side

You've met cortisol; now let us introduce you to leptin and ghrelin. Both are hormones that greatly influence your weight by controlling your appetite. Leptin is secreted in fat tissue and sends a signal to your brain that lets it know you're full. Ghrelin is secreted in the intestinal tract and sends signals indicating that you're hungry.

Leptin and ghrelin are impacted by your sleep habits. Several recent research studies have shown that people who get less than seven hours of sleep per night have elevated ghrelin levels and decreased leptin levels. One of the interesting findings in these studies is that one night of missed or interrupted sleep is enough to see this change in leptin and ghrelin levels. What this means for you is that getting adequate sleep (seven to eight hours minimum), preferably at the same time each night, is essential to keeping leptin and ghrelin on your side. It won't take long to get them regulated, so that you'll soon be overeating less and feeling fewer hunger pangs. This translates to faster belly fat loss without having to do anything other than sleep!

Tool #5: Interval Training

Interval training is simply alternating periods of moderate work with shorter bursts of more intense work. You can apply it to virtually any form of exercise and you can start right where you are, even if you haven't done a bit of exercise in years. The wonderful thing is that your body reacts to the level of exertion you require for your workouts, so beginners can benefit just as much as athletes.

Interval training has been proven to be far more effective than a static (steady paced) workout. In fact, twenty minutes of interval training boosts your metabolism longer than an hour of static exercise!

Interval training works because your body adjusts itself very quickly to your workouts. As you become stronger, your metabolism works less to achieve the same number of reps or the same mileage walked. What this usually means is that people discover they have to work out longer to get the same results. With interval training, you are constantly keeping your body guessing, so your metabolism is never given a chance to adjust and slow down.

This metabolism boost means that you'll burn more calories throughout the day, no matter what you're doing. This allows you to lose fat faster without cutting calories. Another benefit to interval training is that you don't have to spend hours working out. You can spend just twenty or thirty minutes a day on interval training. As you progress, you won't add more time to your workouts, you'll simply adjust the moderate periods to be shorter or more intense and adjust the intense periods to be longer or more difficult, still keeping your total workout time down to twenty or thirty minutes.

These five tools represent the best that all of the new research into fat loss and belly fat have to offer. With these tools, losing that stubborn belly fat is not only possible, it's enjoyable.

Note: *You should talk to your doctor before starting any diet or exercise program, but if you've been diagnosed with type 2 diabetes, it is particularly essential that you let your doctor know your plans (for both diet and exercise) before you get started.*

2

EAT MORE . . . WEIGH LESS

The Belly Fat Diet eating plan allows you to eat as much of the allowed foods as you want, as often as possible. This will keep hunger and cravings at bay, keep your energy high, keep your blood sugar steady, and just make you a whole lot happier and more willing to stick with the plan. However, there are some guidelines to follow.

Eating As Much As You Want Does Not Mean Loading Up Your Plate

Part of reshaping the way you eat is helping your body to be happy with "just enough" food. This means that if you're having chicken breast, a salad, and a baked sweet potato for dinner, you should eat slowly and finish everything before deciding you want more. If you are still hungry, by all means, have another breast or some more veggies. However, your goal should be to eat just until satisfied, not until stuffed. Overstuffing your digestive system is counterproductive to your goals and makes you feel sluggish and uncomfortable.

Learn to Read Your Hunger

As your body adjusts to a healthier diet and your hormones begin to cooperate with you, you'll experience fewer cravings. This usually takes about two weeks. However, you'll have those times when you're hungry, especially in the first few weeks. It's perfectly okay to eat, but for those times when you're standing in front of the fridge, unsure of what it is you want, try satisfying yourself with these foods in this order:

- Try some water—thirst often masks itself as hunger.

- If you're still hungry or know you just crave actual chewing, try a vegetable.

- If you're still hungry, try a fruit.

- If you're still hungry, go for a protein. (You get grains in such limited quantities; don't waste them on a random nosh.)

Why is this order important? For those times when you know you're not truly hungry but are just bored or need something to crunch or chew, trying these foods in this order will keep you from reaching for the higher-calorie, higher-fat, and higher-carbs foods first and eating more than you need to satisfy an urge that isn't really hunger based.

This is not the same situation as planned snacks and meals. This is for eating out of boredom, stress, or nervousness, or what is commonly called emotional eating.

Your Three Limitations: Beef, Grains, and Sweets

There are only three food categories that carry some limitations. They are beef, grains, and sweet treats.

BEEF

Beef is limited because it typically contains a good deal of unhealthful fats, is expensive to buy in healthier, grass-fed varieties, and is usually eaten in fairly large portions. You're limited to one serving per week of steak or roast; the leaner cut the better, trimmed of visible fat. If you don't eat beef, that's all the better.

GRAINS

Most grains are limited because they are easy to overeat, quickly converted to sugar or glucose, and many of them fail to fill you up for very long. You're limited to two servings per day of the grains on the allowed foods list.

SWEETS

Sweet treats are allowed on the eating plan, but they're limited to one per day, and only the sweet treats that are on the Foods List. These are few but tasty. They include frozen fruit pops, nonfat pudding, sorbet, and dark chocolate. Use moderation in your servings of these foods and try to really enjoy them. Eat them at a time when you can focus on how good they taste, rather than eating them mindlessly or in a rush.

It's Not Cheating if It's Part of the Plan!

You're allowed to cheat on this diet.

Once a week, you are allowed to have one thing that you've been craving, missing, waiting for, and doing without. If your true love is pizza, have it. If you've been going through milkshake withdrawal, get one.

Of course, you need to use a bit of sense here. You're not supposed to eat the whole pizza but a slice or two. If you can make it a thin-crust veggie pizza, that would be awesome, but if Hawaiian with extra cheese is the only thing that makes you happy, have it.

Try to choose foods you really love rather than wasting your weekly cheat on something that just shows up. In other words, don't give in to an unplanned slice of mediocre cake at an office party when you've been looking forward to having gourmet ice cream on Saturday.

Going without your favorite foods indefinitely leads to frustration, resentment, and out-of-control cheating. Limiting yourself to your daily sweet and a weekly cheat takes some getting used to at first, but it's much easier than going without altogether. This means you have a much better chance of sticking to the plan until you've reached your goals—and being happier while you do.

What You'll Be Eating on the Belly Fat Diet

Use this guide to help plan your grocery shopping. For the most part, shopping for the Belly Fat Diet is pretty straightforward: shop around the edges of the store, where the produce, meat, seafood, and dairy sections are usually situated. There isn't a whole lot for you in the middle, where the grocery items, convenience foods, and snacks are located.

Fruits and Vegetables

- You can have any fruit you like, as often as you like.

- Fresh is best, but frozen fruits (without syrup or added sugar) are fine for out-of-season fruits or for adding to smoothies and other treats.

- When using fruit as a snack, try to couple it with a protein to lessen the effect on your blood sugar. For example, if you're in the mood for some grapes, have them with a mozzarella stick or a boiled egg.

- All vegetables are allowed on the plan, with the exception of white potatoes and corn. Both are high in starch, which means they're quickly converted to sugar.

- Veggies are best eaten raw, but steaming, roasting, baking, sauté-ing, and stir-frying are perfectly fine.

- As with fruits, fresh veggies are best, but frozen vegetables without butter or cheese sauce added are perfectly acceptable.

- Try to get a wide variety of the power produce items. These are greens that are dark and leafy, and fruits, berries, and veggies that are dark red, orange, or yellow. They have the highest antioxidant and phytonutrient content.

- Canned fruits and veggies are off-limits, as they usually contain fewer vitamins and minerals, less fiber, and a good deal of sugar and additives.

- Buy organic as much as you can afford to. If you're on a tight budget, buy organic fruits and veggies if you'll be eating them raw with peel intact, but you can buy traditional varieties if you'll be peeling or cooking them before you eat.

- You can eat dried figs, dates, cherries, and berries. Choose those without added sugar.

Fish and Seafood

- You can have as much fish and seafood as you like, as long as it isn't breaded, fried, or covered in a cream sauce. It should be steamed, broiled, baked, boiled, or sautéed in a bit of olive or canola oil.

- Try to focus on oily, cold-water fish, as they're the richest in omega-3 fats.

- When choosing any fish, shellfish, and mollusks, fresh is best, even if you'll be freezing it. Make sure it hasn't been thawed from frozen. If it has, you'll need to eat it right away or cook it before you can safely freeze it again.

- Fish from the frozen-food section is okay to buy, as long as it contains no breading, coatings, or sauces.

Meat and Poultry

- You're free to eat chicken breast or ground chicken breast, and turkey breast or ground turkey breast, as often as you like.

- If you want to make sandwiches or salads with these meats, use leftover home-cooked poultry rather than packaged or deli-counter meats. Those contain far too much sodium and too many nitrates and preservatives.

- You're allowed lean cuts of beef steak or beef roast once a week. Rounds and loins are some of the leaner cuts to consider.

- Buy organic, grass-fed meats and poultry if at all possible. You'll avoid the hormones, additives, and other things your body doesn't need.

- When buying ground chicken or turkey, be sure the label says ground breast meat, not just ground chicken or turkey. Regular ground chicken and turkey often include dark meat and skin and contain the same amount of fat as a juicy steak.

Dairy Products

- Dairy products are limited to skim- or reduced-fat milk, almond milk, low-fat or nonfat mozzarella, cottage cheese, and Greek yogurt.

- Limit eggs to free-range or organic.

- Try to limit cow's milk to coffee, cereal, and cooking, rather than using it as a beverage. This will keep your intake down to a healthful level. However, if a cold glass of milk is a real treat for you, go ahead and have it, just keep it down to one glass a day.

- Butter and butter substitutes are off-limits, as are other cheeses.

Grains

- Grains are a good source of fiber, but most of them are converted to sugar quite quickly. They're also one of the easiest foods to overeat. For this reason, grains are limited to two servings per day and you may choose from whole-wheat, whole-grain breads and cereals, brown rice, quinoa, barley, and whole-grain oats.

- When you're choosing your grains, it's a good idea to opt for the most filling choice. A slice of whole grain toast won't stick with you for long, but a bowl of mixed-grain hot cereal will.

- When buying sandwich bread, wraps, or tortillas, make sure they're whole grain. *Whole wheat* does not mean *whole grain*, so read the labels carefully. Also, you want at least six grams of fiber in a slice of bread or it just isn't worth it.

- Make sure to check for high-fructose corn syrup in the ingredients and put the bread back if it's there. Brown rice; quinoa; whole-grain, steel cut oats; and whole, multigrain hot and cold cereals are also okay.

Nuts, Seeds, and Oils

- Nuts and seeds can be an excellent source of healthful fats and fiber, as long as you eat the right ones. Walnuts and almonds are your best choices and should be eaten either raw or roasted without salt or sugar.

- You may also have almond butter or sesame butter that has no trans-fats or sugar added.

- Avocadoes, olive oil, and canola oil are also allowed, as well as pumpkin, sesame, and poppy seeds.

Condiments and Sweet Treats

- Condiments that are not packed with sugars and unhealthful fats are allowed. Ketchup, mayonnaise, and Miracle Whip are off-limits.

- You can enjoy frozen fruit pops with no added sugar, sorbets without added sugar, nonfat pudding and dark chocolate. Limit yourself to one pop, one pudding cup, one scoop of sorbet, or one piece of chocolate the size of a dental floss box per day.

Beverages

- Beverages are limited to water, coffee, and green and black tea.

- You can sweeten your coffee and tea if you must, but limit the sugar in the rest of your diet to accommodate.

- Black coffee is better than coffee with milk, but milk is allowed, while artificial and flavored creamers are not.

- You need to drink a minimum of sixty-four ounces of plain water per day, more if you spend a good deal of time outdoors.

- Juices are not on the diet because they contain little or no fiber, don't fill you up like the whole fruit will, and are easy to overdo. The same is true of flavored waters.

- Sodas are strictly off-limits. Save them for your cheat day if you're really attached to your colas.

- Alcoholic beverages are technically allowed, especially for cooking. Limit yourself to an occasional beer or glass of wine or champagne, though. Avoid mixed drinks.

Other Allowed Foods

- Unsweetened protein powder, honey, agave nectar (as a sugar substitute), all herbs and seasonings, and legumes and beans. (See the Food List for a more complete listing of allowed foods.)

Five Super-Foods You Need to Include on Your Shopping List

All of the foods included on the Belly Fat Diet are extremely healthy and taste great. However, there are some real superstars in the food world: foods that have become known as *super-foods* in the nutritional community. We've highlighted five stars that are easily found in your local store, very affordable, and generally well liked by most people. Keep these on your running grocery list and eat at least one of them each day to give your immune system an extra boost.

BERRIES

Berries are loaded with vitamin C and several of the B vitamins. They're also packed with phytonutrients and antioxidants. The darker the color, the better they are for you. Cranberries, black raspberries, blueberries, and blackberries are all excellent choices.

Kiwi

Kiwi is a nutritional jackpot, but also one of the most affordable super-foods around. Sometimes available for as little as a dime each, these tasty gems are a nutritional bargain. They're packed with vitamin C and fiber and have few calories.

Nuts

Nuts have gotten a bad rap, mostly because people don't understand the difference between healthful fats and unhealthful ones, but also because many of us tend to indulge in varieties that aren't that great for you, such as macadamias and cashews. Nuts provide protein, heart-healthful fats, a ton of insoluble fiber, and a bonus dose of antioxidants. Walnuts and almonds are your healthier choices and you should eat them in as natural a state as possible. Raw is best, roasted okay, too, as long as you skip the salted or honey-roasted types.

Salmon

Salmon is one of the best fish choices for getting omega-3 fatty acids. If salmon is too rich for either your taste buds or your budget, sardines, mackerel, tuna, cod, and other cold-water fish are equally good but more affordable choices.

Sweet Potatoes

These delicious and nutritious vegetables are one of the many orange veggies that make the various super-foods lists. They're very cheap, are packed with antioxidants, have a good amount of protein, and are high in fiber. They also contain a healthy dose of vitamin C. One of the nice things about sweet potatoes is that they satisfy the sweet tooth, too.

SUPPLEMENTS

While the Belly Fat Diet eating plan is filled with foods that are packed with vitamins, minerals, antioxidants, and other essential micronutrients, you'll also be taking a few select supplements that will further nourish your body and help you to lose that belly fat. (It's best to get your doctor's okay before starting on a supplement program, so discuss the list with your doctor before you begin.)

Each morning and evening (or late afternoon), take:

- 1000 mg vitamin C (chewable tablets are fine)
- 1000 mg of a high-quality fish oil supplement
- 1 B vitamin complex (ask your doctor for recommended dosage)

THE BELLY FAT DIET SHOPPING GUIDE

Fruits

- Acai berry—also called Acai fruit
- Apples
- Apricot
- Avocado
- Banana
- Blackberries
- Black raspberries
- Blueberries
- Boysenberries
- Cantaloupe
- Cherries
- Clementines
- Coconut
- Dates
- Figs
- Grapefruit
- Grapes
- Guava

- Honeydew melon
- Honey pomelo
- Jujube—a subtropical fruit
- Lemon
- Lime
- Lingonberries
- Mango
- Nectarines
- Oranges
- Papaya
- Peaches
- Pears
- Persimmon
- Pineapple
- Pitaya or dragon fruit
- Plums
- Pomegranate
- Raspberries
- Star fruit
- Strawberries
- Tangerines
- Ugli fruit
- Watermelon

Vegetables

- Alfalfa sprouts
- Artichoke
- Arugula
- Asparagus
- Bamboo shoots
- Bean sprouts

- Beet greens
- Beets
- Bell peppers
- Bok choy
- Broccoflower
- Broccoli
- Brussels sprouts
- Cabbage
- Carrots
- Cauliflower
- Chard (Swiss and red)
- Chinese cabbage
- Chives
- Collard greens
- Cucumber
- Garlic
- Green onions
- Green peas
- Horseradish
- Kale
- Leeks
- Lettuce (preferably dark, leafy varieties)
- Lima beans
- Mushrooms
- Mustard greens
- Olives
- Onions
- Parsley
- Peppers, preferably orange or red
- Pumpkin
- Sauerkraut

- Shallot
- Snow peas
- Soy beans
- Spinach
- Summer squash
- Sweet potato and yam
- Tomato
- Turnip greens
- Water chestnuts
- Watercress
- Winter squash
- Zucchini

Fish and Seafood

OILY FISH VARIETIES

- Anchovies
- Bloater
- Cacha
- Carp
- Eel
- Herring, fresh
- Hilsa
- Jack fish
- Katla
- Kipper
- Mackerel
- Orange roughy
- Pangas
- Pilchards
- Salmon

- Sardines, in water or olive oil
- Sprats
- Swordfish
- Trout
- Tuna (fresh is best but packed in water is okay, too)
- Whitebait

OTHER GREAT FISH

- Catfish
- Cod
- Flounder
- Haddock
- Skate
- Smelt
- Snapper
- Sole
- Whiting

SHELLFISH, MOLLUSKS, AND MISCELLANEOUS

- Clams
- Crab
- Crawfish
- Lobster
- Octopus
- Oysters
- Prawns
- Scallops
- Shrimp
- Squid

Meats and Poultry

- Chicken breast, skin removed
- Ground chicken breast meat
- Ground turkey breast meat
- Lean beef steaks and roasts, trimmed of all visible fat (limit of one serving per week)
- Turkey breast, skin removed

Dairy Products

- Almond milk
- Eggs
- Greek Yogurt, probiotic if available
- Low-fat or nonfat cottage cheese
- Low-fat or part-skim Mozzarella
- Skim, 1 percent, or 2 percent milk

Grains

- Barley
- Brown rice
- Quinoa
- Whole-grain bread
- Whole-grain hot and cold cereals, no sugar added
- Whole-grain oats
- Whole-grain, whole-wheat flour
- Whole-grain wrap or tortilla

Nuts, Seeds, and Oils

- Almonds
- Almond butter
- Brazil nuts
- Canola oil
- Olive oil
- Pecans
- Pine nuts
- Poppy seeds
- Pumpkin seeds
- Sesame butter
- Sesame seeds
- Walnuts

Other Allowed Foods

- Agave nectar
- Balsamic vinegar
- Black tea
- Coffee
- Bran flakes
- Dried apricots
- Dried blueberries
- Dried cherries
- Dried cranberries
- Dried figs
- Dried peaches
- Dried pineapple
- Flax seed
- Green tea
- Herbs and curry

- Hot sauce
- Honey
- Legumes and beans
- Mustard
- Nori (seaweed paper)
- Psyllium husk
- Rice vinegar
- Soy sauce
- Teriyaki sauce
- Whey or soy protein powder, no sugar

Sweet Treats

- Dark chocolate, minimum 66 percent cacao
- Frozen fruit pops, no sugar
- Nonfat pudding
- Sorbet, no sugar

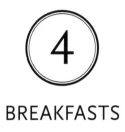

BREAKFASTS

Breakfast Hash

Hash is a combination of meat and vegetables fried in a skillet and is a great way to use leftovers. This recipe uses apple instead of the traditional potato.

- 2 teaspoons olive oil
- 1/4 cup onion, chopped
- 1 cup cooked turkey or chicken, chopped
- 1 tart apple, cored and chopped
- 1/2 teaspoon dried sage
- Sea salt and freshly ground pepper, to taste
- 2 eggs
- 1 tablespoon fresh parsley, chopped

Heat a large nonstick skillet and add olive oil. Add onion and cook until translucent.

In a large bowl, mix the meat, apple, sage, salt, and pepper. Add to onion and stir well.

Cook until meat is heated through and apple has softened.

Make 2 wells in the hash with the back of a spoon and carefully crack in the eggs.

Cover and cook until whites are firm and yolks have cooked to desired consistency. Garnish with parsley.

Serves 2.

Crunchy Granola

Double or triple this recipe and store leftovers in the refrigerator, where it will keep for about a week and a half. If you don't have time to squeeze your own orange juice, use store-bought juice with the pulp.

- 2 tablespoons coconut oil
- 1/4 cup freshly squeezed orange juice
- 1/4 cup honey
- 1 cup oats
- 1 cup raw almonds
- 1 cup raw walnuts
- 1/4 cup sesame seeds
- 1/4 cup flax seeds
- 1 teaspoon ground cinnamon
- 1/2 teaspoon nutmeg
- 1/2 teaspoon powdered ginger
- 1/2 teaspoon sea salt
- 1 tablespoon orange zest

Preheat oven to 350 degrees.

In a small bowl, mix the coconut oil, orange juice, and honey together.

In a large bowl, mix together the remaining ingredients until well combined.

Drizzle the oil mixture over the dry ingredients and stir until evenly coated.

Pack the mixture tightly into a 9 x 13–inch glass baking dish and bake for 30 minutes, until golden brown.

Let cool completely, then break into chunks and store in an airtight container.

Serve with hot or cold low-fat milk or almond milk as a cereal.

Serves 4.

Eggs Benedict

While this might not be the traditional version of eggs Benedict, you'll love this grain-free version that is as good for you as it tastes. Once you try it, you'll never want to go back to the old version!

- 1/2 medium avocado
- 2 tablespoons lemon juice
- 1 clove garlic
- 1 large egg
- 1 tomato slice
- 2 thin slices of turkey breast
- Freshly ground black pepper, to taste

Put the avocado, lemon juice, and garlic in a food processor and process until smooth and creamy.

Poach the egg in a pot of simmering water until done, about 4 minutes.

To serve, place the egg on top of the tomato slice and top with the avocado sauce and turkey.

Season with freshly ground black pepper to taste.

Serves 1.

Fresh Veggie Frittata

You won't miss the cheese with this delicious and filling breakfast. You can use whatever ingredients you have for this recipe—grilled or roasted vegetables add great depth of flavor, as well as nutrition.

- 3 large eggs
- 1 teaspoon almond milk
- 1 tablespoon olive oil
- 1 handful fresh baby spinach leaves
- 1/2 baby eggplant, peeled and diced
- 1/4 small red bell pepper, chopped
- Sea salt and freshly ground pepper, to taste

Preheat the broiler.

Beat the eggs with the almond milk until just combined.

Heat a small nonstick, broiler-proof skillet over medium-high heat. Add the olive oil, followed by the eggs.

Spread the spinach on top of the egg mixture in an even layer and top with the rest of the veggies.

Reduce heat to medium and season with sea salt and freshly ground pepper to taste.

Allow the eggs and vegetables to cook 6–10, minutes until the eggs are firm in the middle.

Place the pan in broiler for about 3–5 minutes. Remove from oven once the top is set and starts to brown. Place a large serving plate over pan, and carefully invert to turn out frittata.

Slice into wedges and serve immediately.

Serves 1.

Green Smoothie

If this nutrient-loaded smoothie isn't sweet enough for you, add half an apple or a small dollop of honey. Feel free to go without the yogurt and, instead, add a 1/2-inch piece of ginger for a completely different taste.

- 1 cucumber, peeled and sliced
- 1/2 lemon, juiced
- 1/2 cup parsley
- 1 stalk celery, sliced
- 1/2 cup plain Greek yogurt
- 1/2 cup cold water

Put all ingredients into blender and mix until frothy.

Serves 1.

Honey and Avocado Smoothie

Avocados are loaded with heart-healthful monounsaturated fats and will definitely fill you up in the morning.

- 1 1/2 cups almond milk
- 1 large avocado
- 2 tablespoons honey

Add all ingredients to your blender and blend until smooth and creamy.

Serve immediately and enjoy!

Serves 2.

Hot Breakfast Rice

This is a great and filling choice for one of your two daily grains.

- 1 cup cooked brown rice
- 1/2 teaspoon cinnamon
- 1/4 cup dried cherries or blueberries
- Pinch of sea salt
- 1/2 cup almond milk
- 1 teaspoon honey

Combine all ingredients in a microwave-safe bowl. Cover and microwave at half power for 1 minute or until heated through.

Serves 2.

Peach and Walnut Breakfast Salad

This inspired dish is light and fresh but feels just a little bit like dessert. You can substitute apples for the pears.

- 1/2 cup low-fat or nonfat cottage cheese, room temperature
- 1 ripe peach, pitted and sliced
- 1/4 cup chopped walnuts, toasted
- 1 teaspoon honey
- 1 tablespoon chopped fresh mint
- Zest of 1 lemon

Put the cottage cheese in a small bowl and top with the peach slices and walnuts.

Drizzle with the honey, then top with the fresh mint and a pinch of lemon zest.

Serve with a spoon.

Serves 1.

Peachy Green Smoothie

You'll get many servings of fruits and vegetables in one delicious drink with this smoothie. It's perfect for days when cooking for yourself is a challenge. Don't forget to use Greek yogurt.

- 1 cup almond milk
- 3 cups kale or spinach
- 1 peeled banana
- 1 peeled orange
- 1 small green apple
- 1 cup frozen peaches
- 1/4 cup vanilla Greek yogurt

Put the ingredients in a blender in the order listed and blend on high until smooth.

Serve and enjoy.

Serves 2.

Savory Breakfast Oats

This savory hot cereal combines the fiber of oats with juicy, sunny flavors. Meanwhile, the herbs and pepper add a little zip.

- 1/2 cup steel cut oats
- 1 cup water
- 1 large tomato, chopped
- 1 medium cucumber, chopped
- 1 tablespoon olive oil
- Fresh chopped parsley or mint for garnish
- Sea salt and freshly ground pepper, to taste

Put the oats and water in a medium saucepan and bring to a boil on high heat.

Stir continuously until water is absorbed, about 15 minutes.

To serve, divide the oatmeal between 2 bowls and top with the tomatoes and cucumber.

Drizzle with olive oil, then top with the herbs.

Season with sea salt and freshly ground pepper to taste.

Serve immediately.

Serves 2.

Spiced Scrambled Eggs

You can enjoy whole eggs on the Belly Fat Diet without worry. Spicy additions not only add flavor but can also help you feel full faster. Enjoy with sliced tomatoes.

- 2 tablespoons olive oil
- 1 small red onion, chopped
- 1 medium green pepper, cored, seeded, and finely chopped
- 1 red Fresno or jalapeño chili pepper, seeded and cut into thin strips
- 3 medium tomatoes, chopped
- Sea salt and freshly ground pepper, to taste
- 1 tablespoon ground cumin
- 1 teaspoon ground coriander
- 4 large eggs, lightly beaten

Heat the olive oil in a large, heavy skillet over medium heat. Add the onion and cook until soft and translucent, about 6–7 minutes.

Add the peppers and continue to cook until soft, another 4–5 minutes.

Add in the tomatoes and season with salt and pepper to taste.

Stir in the cumin and coriander.

Simmer for 10 minutes over medium-low heat.

Add the eggs, stirring them into the mixture to distribute.

Cover the skillet and cook until the eggs are set but still fluffy and tender, about 5–6 minutes more.

Divide between 4 plates and serve immediately.

Serves 4.

Sunrise Smoothie

You can add some bulk to this sweet start to the day by adding ½ cup almond milk or water.

- 1 1/2 cups fresh orange
- 1 cup fresh pineapple
- 1/2 cup sliced mango
- 1/2 banana
- 1 scoop vanilla soy protein powder

Put all ingredients into blender and mix until frothy.

Serves 1.

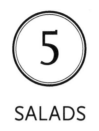

SALADS

Arugula and Artichokes

Arugula, also known as rocket, is a dark leafy green that has a peppery bite. It's very flavorful and has plenty of vitamins A, C, and K, as well as vital phytonutrients. Make this salad with the sweetest cherry tomatoes you can find.

- 4 tablespoons olive oil
- 2 tablespoons aged balsamic vinegar
- 1 teaspoon Dijon mustard
- 1 clove garlic, minced
- 6 cups baby arugula leaves
- 6 oil-packed artichoke hearts, sliced
- 6 oil-cured Kalamata olives, pitted and chopped
- 1 cup cherry tomatoes, sliced in half
- Sea salt and freshly ground pepper, to taste
- 4 fresh basil leaves, thinly sliced

Make the dressing by whisking together the olive oil, balsamic vinegar, Dijon mustard, and garlic until you have a smooth emulsion. Set aside.

Toss the arugula, artichokes, olives, and tomatoes together.

Season with sea salt and freshly ground pepper.

Drizzle the salad with the dressing, garnish with the fresh basil, and serve.

Serves 6.

Cheesy Spinach Salad

Once you've been on the Belly Fat Diet for a while, you won't be as tempted by heavy cheese dressings, soups, etc. Meanwhile, this recipe gives you the creamy texture and taste without the bad fats.

- 2 cups fresh baby spinach leaves
- 1/2 cup nonfat cottage cheese
- 1/2 cup chopped walnuts
- 2 tablespoons honey
- 2 tablespoons vinegar
- 1 teaspoon prepared horseradish
- 1/2 teaspoon Dijon mustard
- Sea salt and freshly ground pepper, to taste

In serving bowl, layer half the spinach and half the cottage cheese and walnuts; repeat in a separate serving bowl.

In small bowl, whisk the remaining ingredients and drizzle over spinach.

Toss to coat evenly.

Serves 2.

Crunchy Chicken Salad

This Asian-inspired salad is hearty, with chicken and healthful vegetables. Serve this salad for lunch or dinner.

- 2 cups baby salad greens
- 1 cup broccoli florets, blanched and rinsed in cold water
- 1 cup cauliflower florets, blanched and rinsed in cold water
- 1/2 cup fresh snow peas, trimmed
- 1/2 red onion, sliced thin
- 1/4 cup soy sauce
- 1 tablespoon cider vinegar
- 1 tablespoon olive oil
- 1 teaspoon honey
- 1 teaspoon sesame seeds, toasted
- 1 cup cooked chicken, cubed

Toss greens, broccoli, cauliflower, snow peas, and onions in a large bowl.

Whisk soy sauce, cider vinegar, olive oil, honey, and sesame seeds in a small bowl and pour over greens.

Toss salad and transfer to plates.

Top each portion with chicken.

Serves 4.

Easy Greek Salad

Avocado, sundried tomatoes, and artichokes, along with crunchy onion and bell peppers, create a satisfying salad loaded with flavor—a nice variation on a classic Greek salad. For best results, use the freshest vegetables you can get your hands on.

- 2 tablespoons balsamic vinegar
- 3 tablespoons olive oil
- 1 teaspoon Greek seasoning
- 1 ripe avocado, peeled and pitted
- 1 red bell pepper, sliced
- 1/4 medium red onion, sliced
- 1 cup black olives, pitted and cut in half
- 2 tomatoes, cut into bite-size pieces
- 1/2 cucumber, halved and sliced
- 1/8 cup sundried tomatoes
- 1/8 cup artichoke hearts
- Freshly ground black pepper, to taste

For the dressing, in a large bowl, whisk together the balsamic vinegar, olive oil, and seasoning.

Combine the rest of the ingredients with the dressing.

Season with freshly ground black pepper to taste.

Let chill, covered, in the refrigerator 30 minutes before serving.

Serves 2.

Endive with Shrimp

This elegant, simple salad makes a delicious lunch entrée. The walnuts provide high levels of omega 3 fatty acids. Serve it with crusty bread and a dry white wine.

- 1/4 cup olive oil
- 1 small shallot, minced
- 1 tablespoon Dijon mustard
- Juice and zest of 1 lemon
- Sea salt and freshly ground pepper, to taste
- 2 cups salted water
- 14 fresh shrimp, peeled and deveined
- 1 head endive
- 1/2 cup tart green apple, diced
- 2 tablespoons toasted walnuts

For the vinaigrette, whisk together the first five ingredients in a small bowl until creamy and emulsified.

Refrigerate for at least 2 hours for best flavor.

In a small pan, boil salted water. Add the shrimp and cook 1–2 minutes, or until the shrimp turn pink. Drain and cool under cold water.

To assemble the salad, wash and break the endive. Place on serving plates and top with the shrimp, green apple, and toasted walnuts.

Drizzle with the vinaigrette before serving.

Serves 4.

Garden Salad with Sardine Filets

Sardines are a super-food, adding vitamin B12, tryptophan, selenium, omega-3 fats, protein, phosphorus, vitamin D, calcium, and vitamin B3. You can serve this salad as a side or a main dish.

- 1/2 cup olive oil
- Juice of 1 lemon
- 1 teaspoon Dijon mustard
- Sea salt and freshly ground pepper, to taste
- 4 medium tomatoes, diced
- 1 large cucumber, peeled and diced
- 1 pound arugula, trimmed and chopped
- 1 small red onion, thinly sliced
- 1 small bunch flat-leaf parsley, chopped
- 4 whole sardine filets packed in olive oil, drained and chopped

For the dressing, whisk together the olive oil, lemon juice, and Dijon mustard, and season with sea salt and freshly ground pepper. Set aside.

In a large bowl, combine all the vegetables with the parsley and toss.

Add the sardine filets on top of the salad.

Drizzle the dressing over the salad just before serving.

Serves 6.

Moroccan Tomato and Roasted Chile Salad

This salad offers bold flavor and big taste. This is a delicious way to get all your veggies in one satisfying dish. Serve with grilled chicken to make this a main dish.

- 2 large green bell peppers
- 1 hot red chili Fresno or jalapeño pepper
- 4 large tomatoes, peeled, seeded, and diced
- 1 large cucumber, peeled and diced
- 1 small bunch parsley, chopped
- 4 tablespoons olive oil
- 1 teaspoon ground cumin
- Juice of 1 lemon
- Sea salt and freshly ground pepper, to taste

Preheat broiler on high. Broil all of the peppers and chilies until the skin blackens and blisters.

Place the peppers and chilies in a paper bag. Seal and set aside to cool.

Combine the rest of the ingredients in a medium bowl and mix well.

Take peppers and chilies out from the bag and remove the skins. Seed and chop the peppers and add them to the salad.

Season with sea salt and freshly ground pepper.

Toss to combine and let sit for 15–20 minutes before serving.

Serves 6.

Peachy Tomato Salad

This is a super-easy summer side dish that is perfect when both tomatoes and peaches are at their best.

- 2 ripe peaches, halved, pitted, and sliced into wedges
- 2 ripe tomatoes, cut into wedges
- 1/2 red onion, thinly sliced
- Sea salt and freshly ground pepper, to taste
- 3 tablespoons olive oil
- 1 tablespoon lemon juice

Toss the peaches, tomatoes, and red onion in a large bowl. Season with sea salt and freshly ground pepper to taste.

Add the olive oil and lemon juice and gently toss.

Serve at room temperature.

Serves 2.

Riviera Tuna Salad

Humble canned tuna becomes something special in this main-dish salad. Garbanzo beans add fiber and protein to this healthy salad.

- 1/4 cup olive oil
- 1/4 cup balsamic vinegar
- 1/2 teaspoon minced garlic
- 1/4 teaspoon dried oregano
- Sea salt and freshly ground pepper, to taste
- 2 tablespoons capers, drained
- 6 cups baby greens
- 4–6 cups baby greens
- 1 can (6-ounce) albacore white tuna packed in water, drained
- 1 cup canned garbanzo beans, rinsed and drained
- 1/4 cup pitted Kalamata olives, quartered
- 2 Roma tomatoes, chopped

To make the vinaigrette, whisk together the olive oil, balsamic vinegar, garlic, oregano, salt, and pepper until emulsified. Stir in the capers.

Refrigerate for up to 6 hours before serving.

Place the baby greens in a salad bowl or on individual plates and top with the tuna, beans, olives, and tomatoes.

Drizzle the vinaigrette over all and serve immediately.

Serves 4.

Tomato and Pepper Salad

Yellow peppers have more nutrients than green peppers and a milder, sweeter flavor. Enjoy this salad with any grilled lean meat or poultry.

- 3 large yellow peppers
- 1/4 cup olive oil
- 1 small bunch fresh basil leaves
- 2 cloves garlic, minced
- 4 large tomatoes, seeded and diced
- Sea salt and freshly ground pepper, to taste

Preheat broiler to high heat and broil the peppers until blackened on all sides.

Remove from heat and place in a paper bag. Seal and allow peppers to cool.

Once cooled, peel the skins off the peppers, then seed and chop them.

Add half of the peppers to a food processor along with the olive oil, basil, and garlic, and pulse several times to make the dressing.

Combine the rest of the peppers with the tomatoes and toss with the dressing.

Season the salad with sea salt and freshly ground pepper.

Allow salad to come to room temperature before serving.

Serves 6.

Warm Fennel, Cherry Tomato, and Spinach Salad

Slightly wilted spinach contrasts nicely with the crunchy fennel in this salad that can serve as a side dish or even a light lunch.

- 4 tablespoons chicken broth
- 4 cups baby spinach leaves
- 10 cherry tomatoes, halved
- Sea salt and freshly ground pepper, to taste
- 1 fennel bulb, sliced
- 1/4 cup olive oil
- Juice of 2 lemons

In a large sauté pan, heat the chicken broth over medium heat. Add the spinach and tomatoes and toss until spinach is wilted. Season with sea salt and freshly ground pepper to taste.

Remove from heat and toss fennel slices in with the spinach and tomatoes. Let the fennel warm in the pan, then transfer to a large bowl.

Drizzle with the olive oil and lemon juice and serve immediately.

Serves 2.

Wilted Kale Salad

Kale can be eaten raw, cooked, or gently sautéed—as it is in this recipe—with a little garlic and olive oil and cherry tomatoes. A nutrient powerhouse, kale is extremely high in vitamin A, vitamin C, and vitamin K. Use a lid to help wilt the kale and keep it in the pan.

- 2 heads kale
- 1 or more tablespoon olive oil
- 2 cloves garlic, minced
- 1 cup cherry tomatoes, sliced
- Sea salt and freshly ground pepper, to taste
- Juice of 1 lemon

Rinse and dry kale. Tear the kale into bite-size pieces.

Heat 1 tablespoon of the olive oil in a large skillet and add the garlic. Cook for 1 minute, then add the kale.

Cook just until wilted, then add the tomatoes.

Cook until tomatoes are softened, then remove from heat.

Place tomatoes and kale in a bowl and season with sea salt and freshly ground pepper.

Drizzle with olive oil and lemon juice, serve, and enjoy.

Serves 4.

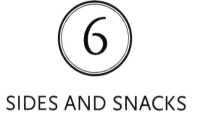

SIDES AND SNACKS

Baked Kale Chips

If you're looking for a crunchy snack to munch on instead of potato chips, you'll love these kale chips. Kale is extremely low in calories, and is one of the most nutrient-dense foods on the planet.

- 2 heads curly leaf kale
- 2 tablespoons olive oil
- Sea salt, to taste

Tear the kale into bite-size pieces. Toss with the olive oil and lay on a baking sheet in a single layer. Sprinkle with a pinch of sea salt.

Bake for 10–15 minutes, until crispy.

Serve or store in an airtight container.

Makes about 4 cups.

Chili Shrimp

This tasty and spicy side is great for potlucks and other fun occasions.

- 1/2 cup olive oil
- 5 cloves garlic, minced
- 1 teaspoon red pepper flakes
- 24 large fresh shrimp, peeled and deveined

- Juice and zest of 1 lemon
- Sea salt and freshly ground pepper, to taste

Heat the oil in a large skillet over medium-high heat. Add the garlic and red pepper flakes and cook for 1 minute.

Add the shrimp and cook an additional 3 minutes, stirring frequently.

Remove from the pan and sprinkle with lemon juice and salt and freshly ground pepper.

Serves 6.

Classic Hummus

Hummus is a creamy and delicious dip that can be served as an appetizer, at a party, or just as a snack. Use hummus in place of mayonnaise on sandwiches.

- 3 cups cooked chickpeas, slightly warmed
- 1/4 cup olive oil
- Juice of 2 lemons
- 2–3 cloves garlic
- 3/4 cup tahini
- Sea salt and freshly ground pepper, to taste
- 1/2 cup pine nuts, toasted (optional)
- 1/4 cup fresh flat-leaf parsley, chopped

Add the chickpeas, olive oil, lemon juice, and garlic to a food processor and puree until smooth.

Add the tahini and continue to blend until creamy. If too thick, a bit of water can be used to thin it.

Season with sea salt and freshly ground pepper to taste.

Add the pine nuts if desired and garnish with chopped parsley.

Serve with fresh veggies or whole-wheat pita wedges.

Serves 6–8.

Curry Onion Dip

The curry flavor of this scrumptious dip will strengthen the longer this dip stands, so make it a day in advance.

- 1 cup raw almonds
- 1 onion, chopped
- 3 tablespoons fresh lime juice
- 3 tablespoons olive oil

- 1 teaspoon curry powder
- 1/2 teaspoon sea salt
- 1/2 teaspoon pepper
- 1/2 teaspoon paprika

Put all ingredients in a food processor and blend until smooth, scraping down sides as needed.

Serve with fresh veggies or whole-wheat pita wedges.

Will keep in refrigerator for up to a week.

Serves 4.

Marinated Olives and Mushrooms

Tangy and salty olives combine with mild button mushrooms to make a marinated treat. These savory morsels are easy to prepare and are especially good to serve at a party. Store in the refrigerator for up to three days, but serve at room temperature.

- 1 pound white button mushrooms
- 1 pound mixed, high-quality olives
- 2 tablespoons fresh thyme leaves
- 1 tablespoon white wine vinegar
- 1/2 tablespoon crushed fennel seeds
- Pinch of chili flakes
- Olive oil, to cover
- Sea salt and freshly ground pepper, to taste

Clean and rinse mushrooms under cold water and pat dry.

Combine all ingredients in a glass jar or other airtight container. Cover with olive oil and season with sea salt and freshly ground pepper.

Shake to distribute the ingredients.

Allow to marinate for at least 1 hour.

Serve at room temperature.

Serves 8.

Mini Lettuce Wraps

Like a Greek salad wrapped in lettuce, this bite-size appetizer is easy to assemble. Swap out the tomatoes, cucumbers, and/or red onion for any vegetables you like. Wraps can be served alone or as part of a larger selection of appetizers.

• 1 tomato, diced	• 1 tablespoon olive oil
• 1 cucumber, diced	• Sea salt and freshly ground pepper, to taste
• 1 red onion, sliced	
• Juice of 1 lemon	• 12 small, intact iceberg lettuce leaves

Combine the tomatoes, cucumber, and onion in a bowl with the lemon juice and olive oil.

Season with sea salt and freshly ground pepper.

Without tearing the leaves, gently fill each leaf with a tablespoon of the veggie mixture. Roll them as tightly as you can and lay them seam side down on a serving platter.

Makes about 1 dozen wraps.

Red Pepper Hummus

You can experiment with the Classic Hummus recipe earlier in this section by adding different herbs, spices, and vegetables. This variation adds a little color and spice.

- 2 cups cooked chickpeas, warmed
- 2 cloves garlic, crushed
- 2 tablespoons lemon juice
- 1/4 cup tahini
- 1/2 cup roasted red sweet pepper, chopped
- Pinch of sea salt
- 1 teaspoon paprika
- 2 tablespoons olive oil

Place all ingredients in food processor and process until smooth.

Serve with fresh veggies or whole-wheat pita wedges.

Will keep in refrigerator for up to four days.

Serves 4–6.

Salted Almonds

These almonds are easy to prepare and make a great snack to serve at a party. High in healthful fats, almonds provide manganese, vitamin E, magnesium, and more.

- 1 cup raw almonds
- 1 egg white, beaten
- 1/2 teaspoon coarse sea salt

Preheat oven to 350 degrees.

Spread the almonds in an even layer on a baking sheet.

Bake for 20 minutes until lightly browned and fragrant.

Coat the almonds with egg white and sprinkle with the salt.

Put back in the oven for about 5 minutes, until they have dried.

Cool completely before serving.

Makes 1 cup.

Savory Mixed Nuts

If you're having trouble giving up on packaged nuts, which often include preservatives, sugar, and too much salt, make this recipe for when you're yearning for nuts.

- 2 cups raw nuts like almonds, walnuts, or pecans
- 1 tablespoon olive oil

- 1 teaspoon seasoned salt (choose your favorite flavor)

Preheat oven to 350 degrees.

Place nuts in a bowl and drizzle with oil.

Toss until evenly coated, then sprinkle with seasoned salt and toss again. Place in a single layer on a large baking sheet and bake for 20 minutes.

Cool completely before serving.

Serves 4.

Shrimp Cocktail

Perfect for game day around the big screen or for whenever you get together with friends. Adjust the ingredients depending on how many people you're expecting.

- 4 tablespoons horseradish
- 2 teaspoons tomato paste
- 1 teaspoon agave nectar
- 2 teaspoons fresh lemon juice
- 12 cooked shrimp, peeled and chilled

Mix horseradish, tomato paste, and agave nectar vigorously.

Squeeze lemon juice into sauce in a small dish.

Serve chilled with shrimp.

Serves 3.

Shrimp Kebabs

Kebabs make a tasty and attractive lunch, and they're almost fat-free.
Shrimp is a good source of protein, and it's high in iron.

- 16–20 count raw shrimp (or prawns)
- 1/2 large fresh pineapple, peeled and top removed
- 1 red bell pepper
- 1 small red onion
- 1 tablespoon rice vinegar
- 2 tablespoons olive oil
- 1 tablespoon chopped fresh oregano
- 6 cherry tomatoes
- Cajun seasoning

Peel and devein the shrimp; drain on paper towels.

Cut the pineapple into 16 chunks of about 1 1/2 inches each.

Remove the stem and seeds from the pepper and cut it into bite-size pieces.

Cut the onion into bite-size pieces.

Mix the rice vinegar, olive oil, and oregano in a small bowl.

Thread the shrimp, pineapple, and vegetables onto skewers and lay them on a baking sheet.

Brush the oil mixture over the kebabs, coating each piece well.

Preheat the grill (or prepare charcoal) and brush the kebabs again with the oil mixture. Just before grilling, dust lightly with Cajun seasoning.

Grill for about 5 minutes on each side, or until the shrimp are browned on the outside and opaque on the inside.

Serves 2.

Spinach Dip

This creamy mixture uses avocado instead of sour cream, but you'll be enjoying this dip too much to even notice the difference. We suggest dipping celery and carrot sticks, but try cucumber, radish, and zucchini as well.

- 1 (10-ounce) package frozen chopped spinach
- 1 ripe avocado
- 1 tablespoon fresh lemon juice
- 1 small onion, chopped
- 1 teaspoon sea salt
- Fresh celery and carrot sticks for dipping

Cook spinach in microwave just until defrosted. Set aside to cool.

Slice avocado in half and remove pit. Scoop flesh into food processor and sprinkle with lemon juice.

Squeeze spinach until almost dry and add to processor with onion and salt. Process for 1 minute until smooth.

Keeps for up to 2 days in refrigerator.

Serves 4.

Sweet Potato Chips

With this recipe you will not miss potato chips, and you won't have to purchase the usually expensive store-bought sweet potato chips. Double or triple the recipe if you want to have this tasty treat on hand for when the munchies hit.

- 1 sweet potato, peeled and cut into 1/4-inch rounds
- 2 teaspoons olive oil
- 1/2 teaspoon Cajun seasoned salt

Preheat oven to 375 degrees.

In a bowl, combine the potato and oil, tossing to coat evenly.

Spread the chips in a single layer on a greased baking sheet and sprinkle evenly with seasoned salt.

Bake for 10 to 12 minutes or until edges of potato chips start to brown.

Serves 1.

Veggie Dip

Here's another delicious dip that doesn't rely on cheese or sour cream for its thick texture and scrumptiousness.

- 1/4 cup fresh parsley leaves, chopped
- 1 red sweet pepper, chopped
- 1/2 cup chopped onion
- 1/4 cup olive oil

- 1 tablespoon fresh lemon juice
- 1 tablespoon tamari sauce
- 1/2 teaspoon black pepper
- Pinch of sea salt
- 1/4 teaspoon cayenne pepper

Put all ingredients in food processor and blend for 1 minute, until thick and smooth.

Store tightly sealed in refrigerator for no more than 5 days.

Serves 4.

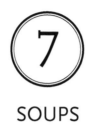

SOUPS

Beans and Chard Soup

This simple soup is rustic and soothing yet nutritionally powerful. Serve it with a green salad and a slice of whole-grain bread.

- 1 cup dried pinto beans, soaked overnight
- 1/4 cup olive oil
- 1 medium onion, diced
- 4 cups chicken stock or water

- 2 cups chard or Swiss chard, sliced, tough stems removed
- 1 medium tomato, diced
- 1/2 teaspoon thyme
- Sea salt and freshly ground pepper, to taste

Drain and rinse the soaked pinto beans.

Heat the olive oil in a stockpot over medium heat.

Sauté the onion for 5–8 minutes, or until tender and translucent.

Add the remaining ingredients, including the pinto beans, and heat to a simmer.

Cover and cook on low for 1–2 hours, or until the beans are tender, but not falling apart.

Serves 6.

Traditional Chicken Soup

A tasty dose of vitamins, chicken soup is a delicious way to consume nutrients and stay healthy. Spring asparagus, peas, spinach, and chives add freshness to this chicken soup.

- 1 (32-ounce) carton chicken broth
- 1 (10-ounce) package frozen peas and pearl onions
- 1 carrot, peeled and sliced thin
- 1 bunch asparagus, trimmed and cut into 1-inch pieces
- 1 cup fresh spinach, chopped
- 1/2 teaspoon dried marjoram
- 1/2 teaspoon sea salt
- 1/4 teaspoon freshly ground pepper
- 1/4 teaspoon ground nutmeg
- 1 cup cooked chicken, diced
- 1/4 cup cold water
- 2 tablespoons arrowroot
- 1/2 cup chives, chopped

Bring broth to a boil in a soup pot over high heat.

Add peas and carrot and reduce heat to a simmer. Cook for 2 minutes and add asparagus, spinach, and seasonings. Cook for 5 minutes, or until vegetables are tender.

Increase heat and add chicken.

In small bowl, combine arrowroot with cold water and mix until thoroughly blended.

Add to the hot soup, stirring until slightly thickened. Remove from heat and stir in chives just before serving.

Serves 4.

Cold Cucumber Soup

Nothing's more refreshing on a hot day than this classic soup. Serve it with a salad for a light lunch or dinner.

- 2 seedless cucumbers, peeled and cut into chunks
- 2 cups plain Greek yogurt
- 1/2 cup mint, finely chopped
- 2 garlic cloves, minced
- 2 cups chicken broth or vegetable stock
- 3 teaspoons fresh dill
- 1 tablespoon tomato paste
- Sea salt and freshly ground pepper, to taste

Puree the cucumbers, yogurt, mint, and garlic in a food processor or blender.

Add the chicken broth or vegetable stock, dill, tomato paste, salt, and pepper, and blend to incorporate.

Refrigerate for at least 2 hours before serving.

Serves 4.

Lentil Soup with Spinach

Lentils are similar to beans as far as flavor and nutrients go, but they have one distinct advantage when it comes to preparation: they cook much faster than beans. While rich and creamy, they are also very low in calories.

- 1 teaspoon olive oil
- 1 cup onion, chopped
- 1 1/2 cups lentils
- 1 tablespoon curry powder
- 6 cups water
- 12 ounces fresh spinach

Heat the olive oil and sauté the onion.

Add the lentils and curry powder and stir.

Add the water and cook until lentils are tender, about 15–20 minutes.

Add the spinach and stir until wilted.

Serve with toasted whole-wheat bread and a green salad.

Serves 6.

Quick Rotisserie Chicken Soup

You can purchase rotisserie chickens fully cooked at most grocery stores. Read the label and make sure the ingredients list is as simple as possible, with no disallowed items.

- 1 fully cooked and seasoned rotisserie chicken
- 1 cup peeled baby carrots
- 1/2 cup chopped celery
- 1 cup fresh spinach leaves
- 4 cups chicken stock
- 2 tablespoons chopped fresh parsley

Cut chicken in half lengthwise so that it will easily be covered by stock. Place in a large, heavy stockpot.

Add the rest of the ingredients, except for the parsley.

Bring to a boil, lower heat to a simmer, cover, and cook for 45 minutes.

Remove chicken, pull all meat from bones, discarding the skin.

Shred or chop chicken, return to pot to reheat, and serve with a sprinkling of fresh parsley.

Serves 4.

Shrimp Soup with Leeks and Fennel

The flavors of leeks, fennel, garlic, and shrimp are featured in this elegant soup. Soup like this is low in calories yet filling, and provides several servings of vegetables. You can substitute scallops for the shrimp if you prefer.

- 2 tablespoons olive oil
- 3 stalks celery, chopped
- 1 leek, both whites and light green parts, sliced
- 1 medium fennel bulb, trimmed and chopped
- 1 clove garlic, minced
- Sea salt and freshly ground pepper, to taste
- 1 tablespoon fennel seeds
- 4 cups vegetable or chicken broth
- 1 pound medium shrimp, peeled and deveined
- 2 tablespoons light cream
- Juice of 1 lemon

Heat the oil in a large Dutch oven over medium heat.

Add the celery, leek, and fennel, and cook for about 15 minutes, until vegetables are browned and very soft.

Add the garlic and season with sea salt and freshly ground pepper to taste.

Add the fennel seed and stir.

Add the broth and bring to a boil, then reduce to a simmer and cook about 20 more minutes.

Add the shrimp to the soup and cook until just pink, about 3 minutes.

Add the cream and lemon juice and serve immediately.

Serves 6.

Spinach and Brown Rice Soup

This recipe calls for a lot of spinach; however, cooking the spinach reduces it significantly. Note that this meal counts as one of your two allowed daily grains.

- 1 tablespoon olive oil
- 1 large onion, chopped
- 2 cloves garlic, minced
- 3 pounds fresh spinach leaves, stems removed and leaves chopped
- 8 cups chicken broth
- 1/2 cup long-grain brown rice
- Sea salt and freshly ground pepper, to taste

Heat the olive oil in a large Dutch oven over medium heat and add the onion and garlic. Cook until the onions are soft and translucent, about 5 minutes.

Add the spinach and stir. Cover the pot and cook the spinach until wilted, about 3 more minutes.

Using a slotted spoon, remove the spinach and onions from the pot, leaving the liquid.

Put the spinach mixture in a food processor or blender and process until smooth, then return to the pot.

Add the chicken broth and bring to a boil.

Add the rice, reduce heat, and simmer until rice is cooked, about 45 minutes.

Season with sea salt and pepper to taste.

Serve hot.

Serves 6.

Tomato Soup

This version of tomato soup is subtly flavored with the classic spices of Morocco—paprika, ginger, cumin, and cinnamon. Cooked tomatoes are a great source of lycopene.

- 2 tablespoons olive oil
- 1 large onion, coarsely chopped
- 8 large tomatoes, seeded and coarsely chopped
- 1 teaspoon paprika
- 1 teaspoon finely chopped fresh ginger
- 1 teaspoon ground cumin
- 2 cups chicken broth
- 1 cinnamon stick
- 1 teaspoon honey
- Sea salt and freshly ground pepper, to taste
- Juice of 1 lemon
- 1 small bunch parsley, chopped
- 2 tablespoons chopped cilantro

Heat a large Dutch oven over medium-high heat. Add the olive oil and onion and cook until soft and translucent.

Add the tomatoes and the seasonings and stir.

Pour in the chicken broth and add the cinnamon stick and honey. Simmer for 15 minutes and puree the soup in a food processor or blender, (remove the cinnamon stick for this step and return it when done).

Pour back into the pot and season with sea salt and freshly ground pepper to taste.

Stir in the lemon juice and serve garnished with the cilantro and parsley.

Serves 6.

White Bean, Cherry Tomato, and Kale Soup

This soup is as inexpensive as it is filling and nutritious. Substitute vegetable stock if you want to make this completely vegetarian.

- 2 tablespoons olive oil
- 1 small onion, chopped
- 2 cloves garlic, minced
- 1 bunch Tuscan kale, torn into bite-size pieces
- 6 cups chicken or vegetable broth
- 2 pints cherry tomatoes, halved
- 2 cans white beans of your choice, drained and rinsed
- Sea salt and freshly ground pepper, to taste
- Freshly grated Parmesan cheese for serving

Heat the oil in a large soup pot or Dutch oven over medium heat. Add the onions and cook for 5 minutes, or until soft and translucent.

Add the garlic and cook for 1 more minute.

Add the kale and stir until well coated with the oil.

Add the broth and bring to a boil on high heat.

Reduce heat to low and simmer for 15 minutes, until kale is softened.

Add the tomatoes and beans and simmer for 5 more minutes.

Season with sea salt and freshly ground pepper to taste.

To serve, ladle into bowls and sprinkle with freshly grated Parmesan cheese.

Serves 4.

SANDWICHES AND WRAPS

Avocado and Asparagus Wraps

Avocados are not just for guacamole—they are a great addition to your diet because of their healthy fats. Use mashed avocados in place of mayonnaise in salads, sandwiches, and wraps. This wrap is served warm, and could also be served as a light meal or snack.

- 12 spears asparagus
- 1 ripe avocado, mashed slightly
- Juice of 1 lime
- 2 cloves minced garlic
- 2 cups brown rice, cooked and chilled
- 3 tablespoons Greek yogurt
- Sea salt and freshly ground pepper, to taste
- 3 (8-inch) whole-grain tortillas
- 1/2 cup chopped cilantro
- 2 tablespoons diced red onion

Steam asparagus in microwave or stove-top steamer until tender.

Mash the avocado, lime juice, and garlic in a medium-size mixing bowl.

In a separate bowl, mix the rice and yogurt.

Season both mixtures with sea salt and freshly ground pepper to taste.

Heat the tortillas in a dry nonstick skillet.

Spread each tortilla with the avocado mixture and top with the rice, cilantro, and onion, followed by the asparagus.

Fold both sides of the tortilla up and roll tightly to close. Cut in half diagonally before serving.

Serves 6.

Chicken Sandwich

If you're looking for sandwiches while on the Belly Fat Diet, you have to pay particular attention to the bread you use—see the section on selecting whole-grain breads. That's okay, though, because with this recipe, you don't need the bread anyway.

- 2 tablespoons olive oil
- 2 free-range, organic chicken breasts
- Freshly ground black pepper, to taste
- 4 large lettuce leaves, intact and untorn
- 2 tablespoons mustard
- Lemon juice, for seasoning
- 1 tomato, seeded and diced

In a large skillet, heat the oil on medium-high heat. Add the chicken breasts and sear until browned.

Flip over and finish cooking, making sure the chicken is brown and crispy on both sides.

Season with freshly ground black pepper to taste.

When the chicken is cool, slice into strips.

Spread each lettuce leaf with mustard, being careful not to tear the leaves. Add the chicken.

Season with lemon juice if desired.

Top with tomato and fold into wraps to serve.

Serves 2.

Cucumber Basil Sandwiches

The addition of basil adds antioxidants and flavor to this hummus sandwich. The skin and seeds of the cucumber contain many nutrients, so don't remove them. Make it an open-face sandwich to further reduce the carbohydrates and calories, if you'd like.

- 4 slices whole-grain bread
- 1/4 cup hummus
- 1 large cucumber, thinly sliced
- 4 whole basil leaves

Spread the hummus on 2 slices of bread and layer the cucumbers on them.

Top with the basil leaves and close the sandwiches.

Press down lightly and serve immediately.

Serves 2.

Grilled Chicken Salad Wrap

Tender and juicy grilled chicken topped with fresh vegetables and wrapped in a whole-grain tortilla makes a filling and hearty meal. Serve this with celery and carrot sticks on the side for crunch instead of salty chips.

- 1 boneless, skinless chicken breast
- Sea salt and freshly ground pepper, to taste
- 1 cup baby spinach
- 1 roasted red pepper, sliced
- 1 tomato, chopped
- 1/2 small red onion, thinly sliced
- 1/2 small cucumber, chopped
- 4 tablespoons olive oil
- Juice of 1 lemon
- 1 whole-grain tortilla

Preheat a gas or charcoal grill to medium-high heat.

Season the chicken breast with sea salt and freshly ground pepper and grill until cooked through, about 7–8 minutes per side.

Allow chicken to rest for 5 minutes before slicing into strips.

While the chicken is cooking, put all the chopped vegetables into a medium-size mixing bowl and season with sea salt and freshly ground pepper.

Chop the chicken into cubes and add to salad.

Add the olive oil and lemon juice and toss well.

Place the mixture on a tortilla and wrap. Serve immediately.

Serves 1.

Mediterranean Tuna Salad Sandwiches

Usually loaded with high-fat mayonnaise, tuna salad is not often thought of as a healthy staple. This version is made with Greek yogurt and roasted peppers, adding flavor and moisture without a lot of fat. You can also enjoy the tuna salad without the bread, if you prefer.

- 1 can (6-ounce) albacore white tuna packed in water, drained
- 1 roasted red pepper, diced
- 1/2 small red onion, diced
- 10 Kalamata olives, finely chopped
- 1/4 cup plain Greek yogurt
- 1 tablespoon fresh parsley, chopped
- Juice of 1 lemon
- Sea salt and freshly ground pepper, to taste
- 4 whole-grain pieces of bread

In a small bowl, combine all the ingredients except the bread, and mix well.

Season with sea salt and freshly ground pepper to taste.

Toast the bread or warm in a pan.

Make the sandwich and serve immediately.

Serves 2.

Spinach and Mushroom Pita

This easy-to-put-together pita pocket makes a light and healthy lunch option. All of the ingredients in the sandwich can also be used in salads, so stock up your refrigerator produce drawer!

- 2 cups baby spinach leaves
- 1 small red onion, thinly sliced
- 1/2 cup sliced button mushrooms
- 1/2 cup alfalfa sprouts
- 1 tomato, chopped
- 1/2 small cucumber
- 2 tablespoons olive oil
- Juice of 1 lemon
- Sea salt and freshly ground pepper, to taste
- 2 whole-grain pita pockets

Combine all the vegetables, olive oil, and lemon juice in a bowl and season with sea salt and freshly ground pepper to taste.

Toss the salad until well mixed.

Stuff the vegetable mixture into the pita pockets and serve immediately.

Serves 2.

Tuna-Stuffed Avocado

This vibrant version of tuna salad has no mayonnaise. Add chopped green onions or capers for variety. Make a wrap with this recipe or eat it out of the avocado shells.

- 1 avocado, halved and pitted
- 2 teaspoons fresh lemon juice
- 1 can (6-ounce) albacore white tuna packed in water, drained
- 1 stalk celery, thinly sliced
- 2 tablespoons fresh cilantro or parsley, chopped
- 1 teaspoon olive oil
- Pinch of cayenne pepper

Scoop the avocado flesh into a large bowl and chop roughly; reserve the shells.

Sprinkle flesh with lemon juice.

Flake the tuna into the avocado and toss. Add celery, cilantro, olive oil, and cayenne, and toss to combine.

Fill the avocado shells with the tuna mixture and serve.

Serves 2.

Turkey Patties

Missing hamburgers? Try this simple recipe using ground turkey instead of beef. To make the bread crumbs, use a piece of whole-grain bread left out overnight.

- 1 egg, lightly beaten
- 1/2 cup whole-grain bread crumbs
- 1/3 cup finely chopped celery
- 1/3 cup finely chopped onion
- 2 teaspoons dried parsley
- 1 teaspoon dried oregano
- 1/2 teaspoon sea salt
- 1/4 teaspoon freshly ground pepper
- 1 pound lean ground turkey breast
- 2 teaspoons Worcestershire sauce
- 1 tablespoon olive oil

In a bowl, combine the egg, crumbs, celery, onion, and seasonings. Mix well. Crumble the turkey into the bowl and mix well to combine.

Form into 4-inch patties, 1-inch thick.

Brush both sides with Worcestershire sauce.

Heat frying pan over medium heat, add oil, and cook patties for 5 minutes on each side.

Serves 4.

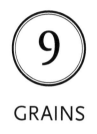

GRAINS

Apple Couscous with Curry

This dish has a complex variety of sweet and savory flavors. The light and fluffy couscous is stuffed with crunchy chopped nuts, but feel free to substitute walnuts or pistachios for the pecans.

- 2 teaspoons olive oil
- 2 leeks, white parts only, sliced
- 1 Granny Smith apple, diced
- 2 cups cooked whole-wheat couscous
- 2 tablespoons curry powder
- 1/2 cup chopped pecans

Heat the olive oil in a large skillet on medium heat and add leeks. Cook until soft and tender, about 5 minutes.

Add diced apple and cook until soft.

Add couscous and curry powder, stir to combine.

Remove from heat, mix in nuts, and serve.

Serves 4.

Brown Rice with Apricots, Cherries, and Toasted Pecans

Brown rice is a great source of fiber and combines easily with lots of other healthful additions. The dried apricots and cherries add tartness to this dish, while the pecans add crunch and extra flavor. Feel free to use walnuts or almonds in place of the pecans.

- 2 tablespoons olive oil
- 2 green onions, sliced
- 1/2 cup brown rice
- 1 cup chicken stock
- 4–5 dried apricots, chopped
- 2 tablespoons dried cherries
- 2 tablespoons toasted and chopped pecans
- Sea salt and freshly ground pepper, to taste

Heat the olive oil in a medium saucepan and add the green onions.

Sauté for 1–2 minutes and add the rice. Stir to coat in oil and add the stock.

Bring to a boil, reduce heat, and cover. Simmer for 50 minutes.

Add the apricots, cherries, and pecans, and cover again for 10 more minutes.

Fluff with a fork to mix the fruit into the rice, season with sea salt and freshly ground pepper, and serve.

Serves 2.

Couscous with Apricots

This vegetarian dish is as pretty as it is delicious. Adding dried fruits and nuts adds a nutritious boost. Serve with chicken or eat it by itself.

- 2 tablespoons olive oil
- 1 small onion, diced
- 1 cup couscous
- 2 cups water or broth
- 1/2 cup dried apricots, soaked in water overnight
- 1/2 cup slivered almonds or pistachios
- 1/2 teaspoon dried mint
- 1/2 teaspoon dried thyme

Heat the olive oil in a large skillet over medium-high heat. Add the onion and cook until translucent and soft.

Stir in the couscous and cook for 2–3 minutes.

Add the water or broth, cover, and cook for 8–10 minutes until the water is mostly absorbed.

Remove from the heat and let stand for a few minutes.

Fluff with a fork and fold in the apricots, nuts, mint, and thyme.

Serves 4.

Crunchy Pea and Barley Salad

Quick-cooking barley doesn't take long to prepare and is loaded with fiber and antioxidants. Served on its own, this salad makes a filling vegetarian meal, but it also works as a side dish.

- 2 cups water
- 1 cup quick-cooking barley
- 2 cups sugar snap pea pods
- Small bunch flat-leaf parsley, chopped
- 1/2 small red onion, diced
- 2 tablespoons olive oil
- Juice of 1 lemon
- Sea salt and freshly ground pepper, to taste

Bring water to boil in a saucepan. Stir in the barley and cover.

Simmer for 10 minutes until all water is absorbed, and then let stand about 5 minutes covered.

Rinse the barley under cold water and combine it with the peas, parsley, onion, olive oil, and lemon juice.

Season with sea salt and freshly ground pepper to taste.

Serves 4.

Cumin-Scented Lentils with Rice

This classic Lebanese dish, called Megadarra, pairs well with chicken or fish.

- 1/4 cup olive oil
- 1 medium onion, thinly sliced
- 1 tablespoon ground cumin
- 1 cup green lentils
- 2 cups water, divided
- 3/4 cup long-grain rice, rinsed
- 2 bay leaves
- Sea salt and freshly ground pepper, to taste

Heat a large saucepan over medium heat. Add the olive oil and onion, and sauté for 10 minutes, until soft and translucent.

Add the cumin and stir to incorporate.

Add the lentils and stir to coat in the oil.

Add 1 cup water, bring to a boil, and reduce to a simmer. Simmer for 15 minutes, until most of the water has been absorbed.

Add the rice to the pot, along with 1 cup water and the bay leaves, and bring to a boil.

Reduce heat, cover, and simmer for 15–20 more minutes, checking periodically and adding water to prevent rice or lentils from becoming scorched.

When both the rice and lentils are tender and cooked through, stir and season with sea salt and freshly ground pepper.

Remove the bay leaves and serve immediately.

Serves 2.

Herbed Barley

Barley was one of the first cultivated grains from the Fertile Crescent, a region that encompasses modern Israel, Iraq, Syria, Lebanon, and Palestine. It's a good source of dietary fiber. Serve this dish with roasted chicken.

- 2 tablespoons olive oil
- 1/2 cup diced onion
- 1/2 cup diced celery
- 1 carrot, peeled and diced
- 3 cups water or chicken broth
- 1 cup barley
- 1 bay leaf
- 1/2 teaspoon thyme
- 1/2 teaspoon rosemary
- 1/4 cup walnuts or pine nuts
- Sea salt and freshly ground pepper, to taste

Heat the olive oil in a medium saucepan over medium-high heat. Sauté the onion, celery, and carrot over medium heat until they are tender.

Add the water or chicken broth, barley, and seasonings, and bring to a boil. Reduce the heat and simmer for 25 minutes, or until tender.

Stir in the nuts and season to taste.

Serves 4.

Quinoa and Broccoli

Originally from the Andes, quinoa is a fast and easy-to-cook starch that is extremely healthy. It's high in manganese, magnesium, protein, and more. Be sure to rinse quinoa before cooking, otherwise it may have a bitter flavor.

- 2 tablespoons olive oil
- 1 cup broccoli florets
- 2 cups cooked quinoa
- Zest of 1 lemon
- Sea salt and freshly ground pepper, to taste

Heat the oil in a large skillet. Add the broccoli and cook until soft, about 3 minutes.

Take off heat and add the quinoa and lemon zest. Season with salt and pepper and serve.

Serves 4.

Rice and Lentils

Here, brown rice is used instead of the classic white rice. This version has a touch of sweetness from the caramelized onions. Cook the onions very slowly, stirring frequently so they caramelize and don't burn.

- 2 cups green or brown lentils
- 1 cup brown rice
- 5 cups water or chicken stock
- 1/2 teaspoon sea salt
- 1/2 teaspoon freshly ground pepper
- 1/2 teaspoon dried thyme
- 1/4 cup olive oil
- 3 onions, peeled and sliced

Place the lentils and rice in a large saucepan with water or chicken stock. Bring to a boil, cover, and simmer for 20–25 minutes, or until almost tender.

Add the seasonings and cook an additional 20–30 minutes, or until the rice is tender and the water is absorbed.

In another saucepan, heat the olive oil over medium heat. Add the onions and cook very slowly, stirring frequently, until the onions become browned and caramelized, about 20 minutes.

To serve, ladle the lentils and rice into bowls and top with the caramelized onions.

Serves 4.

Rice Pilaf

Pilaf is a type of rice dish that pairs well with fish and poultry. This dish is seasoned traditionally with cinnamon and raisins, but you can omit them if you prefer.

- 2 tablespoons olive oil
- 1 medium onion, diced
- 1/4 cup pine nuts
- 1 1/2 cups long-grain rice
- 2 1/2 cups chicken stock
- 1 cinnamon stick
- 1/4 cup raisins
- Sea salt and freshly ground pepper, to taste

Heat the olive oil in a large saucepan over medium heat. Sauté the onions and pine nuts for 6–8 minutes, or until the pine nuts are golden and the onion is translucent.

Add the rice and sauté for 2 minutes until lightly brown.

Pour the chicken stock into the pan and bring to a boil.

Add the cinnamon and raisins.

Lower the heat, cover the pan, and simmer for 15–20 minutes, or until the rice is tender and the liquid is absorbed. Season with salt and pepper to taste.

Remove from the heat and fluff with a fork.

Serves 6.

Skillet Bulgur with Kale and Tomatoes

Originally from the Middle East, bulgur is high in protein and fiber. A great side dish, it can be served with roast chicken or fish.

- 2 tablespoons olive oil
- 2 cloves garlic, minced
- 1 bunch kale, trimmed and cut into bite-size pieces
- Juice of 1 lemon
- 2 cups cooked bulgur wheat
- 1 pint cherry tomatoes, halved
- Sea salt and freshly ground pepper, to taste

Heat the olive oil in a large skillet over medium heat. Add the garlic and sauté for 1 minute.

Add the kale leaves and stir to coat. Cook for 5 minutes until leaves are cooked through and thoroughly wilted.

Add the lemon juice, followed by the bulgur and tomatoes.

Season with sea salt and freshly ground pepper, and serve.

Serves 2.

POULTRY

Arroz con Pollo

This dish is easy to prepare and can be adapted to your taste. Add more vegetables such as artichokes or peas to boost fiber and decrease calories.

- 4 tablespoons olive oil
- 1 chicken, cut up
- Sea salt and freshly ground pepper, to taste
- 3 sweet red peppers, coarsely chopped
- 1 onion, chopped
- 2 garlic cloves, minced
- 2 1/2 cups chicken stock
- 1 (14-ounce) can diced tomatoes, drained
- 1 tablespoon paprika
- 1 cup brown rice
- 1/4 cup flat-leaf parsley, chopped

Heat the olive oil in a large skillet on medium-high heat. Place the chicken in the pan and cook it 8–10 minutes, or until lightly browned on both sides.

Transfer the chicken to an oven-safe dish and keep warm in the oven on the lowest setting.

Add sea salt and freshly ground pepper to taste.

Add the sweet peppers, onion, and garlic to the skillet, and cook, stirring frequently, until tender.

Heat the chicken stock in the microwave or a saucepan until simmering. Add the chicken stock, tomatoes, and paprika to the pan.

Stir in the rice and place the chicken pieces on top.

Simmer with the lid on for 20–30 minutes, or until the liquid is absorbed and the rice is tender.

Garnish with parsley.

Serve with a green salad or tomato and red onion salad.

Serves 6.

Chicken Fried Rice for One

This hearty stir-fried rice dish is a good way to use up leftover rice and chicken. Cold rice is best for stir-fry dishes because the starch enables the rice to stay firm.

- 1 teaspoon canola oil
- 1 carrot, thinly sliced
- 1/4 cup onions, slivered
- 1/2 cup cooked chicken, shredded
- 1/4 cup frozen peas

- 1 tablespoon soy sauce
- 1 cup cold, cooked brown rice
- A few drops toasted sesame oil
- 1/4 teaspoon red pepper flakes

Heat a medium-size frying pan over medium heat, add the oil, and cook the carrots for 1 minute.

Add the onion and stir-fry for 2 minutes.

Add chicken, peas, and soy sauce, and continue stir-frying for another minute.

Crumble the rice into the pan, separating it into individual grains. Cook, stirring, until heated through.

Sprinkle with sesame oil and red pepper, and serve.

Serves 1.

Chicken Marsala

The secret to this classic is to pound the chicken breasts thin between 2 pieces of wax paper so they cook quickly and evenly. Small servings of meat and large portions of vegetables are easy to achieve with this entrée.

- 1/4 cup olive oil
- 4 boneless, skinless chicken breasts, pounded thin
- Sea salt and freshly ground pepper, to taste
- 1/4 cup flour
- 1/2 pound mushrooms, sliced
- 1 cup Marsala
- 1 cup chicken broth
- 1/4 cup flat-leaf parsley, chopped

Heat the olive oil in a large skillet on medium-high heat. Salt and pepper the chicken breasts and dredge them in flour.

Sauté them in the olive oil until golden brown.

Transfer to an oven-safe plate and keep warm in the oven on low.

Sauté the mushrooms in the original pan. Add the wine and chicken broth and bring to a simmer.

Simmer for 10 minutes, or until the sauce is reduced and thickened slightly.

Return the chicken to the pan and cook it in the sauce for 10 minutes.

Transfer to a serving dish and sprinkle with the parsley.

Serves 4.

Chicken Stir-Fry

Chicken and rice makes a quick one-dish meal. Use broccoli instead of celery to add more nutrition, if you prefer.

- 1 tablespoon canola oil
- 1/2 onion, sliced and quartered
- 1 stalk celery, sliced diagonally
- 1 clove garlic, minced
- 1 tablespoon soy sauce
- 1 cup cold, cooked brown rice
- 1/2 cup cooked chicken, cubed

Heat a wok or large nonstick skillet over medium-high heat. Add oil, then cook onion, celery, and garlic, stirring constantly, for 1 minute.

Add soy sauce and stir well.

Add rice and chicken, stirring to break up and color rice evenly.

Cook until heated through and serve.

Serves 2.

Chicken Tagine with Olives

Tagine is a traditional Moroccan stew. This version gets its bright color from saffron and turmeric. Use a combination of purple and green pitted olives if you can find them. Olives are a good source of vitamin E.

- 1 teaspoon ground ginger
- 1/2 teaspoon ground cumin
- 1/2 teaspoon paprika
- 1/2 teaspoon turmeric
- Pinch of saffron threads
- 1 clove garlic, minced
- 1 whole chicken
- 2 medium onions, thinly sliced
- 1/2 cup finely chopped flat-leaf parsley
- 1/2 cup finely chopped fresh cilantro
- 1 cinnamon stick
- 3 cups water
- 2 tablespoons olive oil
- 1 tablespoon butter
- Juice and zest of 1 lemon
- 1 cup green or purple olives (or a combination of both)
- Sea salt and freshly ground pepper, to taste

Combine the spices and garlic in a small bowl.

Pat the chicken dry, brush the spices over the chicken, and massage it in with your fingers, including in the cavity.

Place the chicken in a large stew pot or Dutch oven.

Add the onions, parsley, cilantro, and cinnamon stick to the pot along with the water.

Bring the water to a boil and add the olive oil, butter, and lemon zest and juice.

Cover and simmer for 1–2 hours, or until the chicken is tender and the sauce has reduced and thickened slightly.

Remove the lid and simmer an additional 15 minutes. Season with salt and pepper to taste.

Add the olives immediately before serving.

Serves 6.

Citrus Chicken with Pecan Wild Rice

This combination of sunny orange, healthy nuts, and wild rice fits well with the Belly Fat Diet. Wild rice is a good source of fiber, zinc, iron, vitamin B1, vitamin B2, vitamin B3, and vitamin B9.

- 4 boneless, skinless chicken breasts
- Sea salt and freshly ground pepper, to taste
- 2 tablespoons olive oil
- Juice and zest of 1 orange
- 2 cups wild rice, cooked
- 2 green onions, sliced
- 1 cup pecans, toasted and chopped

Season chicken breasts with sea salt and freshly ground pepper.

Heat a large skillet over medium heat. Add oil and sear the chicken until browned on 1 side.

Flip the chicken and brown other side.

Add orange juice to the skillet and let cook down.

In a large bowl, combine the rice, onions, pecans, and orange zest.

Season with sea salt and freshly ground pepper to taste.

Serve the chicken alongside the rice and a green salad for a complete meal.

Serves 4.

Grilled Chicken and Vegetables with Lemon-Walnut Sauce

This grilled chicken and vegetable dish gets a boost from a rich pureed walnut sauce. Other vegetables such as artichokes, carrots, eggplant, or endive can be used in place or in addition to the zucchinis and asparagus.

- 1 cup chopped walnuts, toasted
- 1 small shallot, very finely chopped
- 1/2 cup olive oil, plus more for brushing
- Juice and zest of 1 lemon
- 4 boneless, skinless chicken breasts
- Sea salt and freshly ground pepper, to taste
- 2 zucchinis, sliced diagonally 1/4-inch thick
- 1/2 pound asparagus
- 1 red onion, sliced 1/3-inch thick
- 1 teaspoon Italian seasoning

Preheat a grill to medium-high heat.

While you're waiting for it to heat up, make the walnut sauce by putting the walnuts, shallots, olive oil, and lemon juice and zest in a food processor and processing until smooth and creamy.

Season the chicken with sea salt and freshly ground pepper, and grill on an oiled grate until cooked through, about 7–8 minutes a side or until an instant-read thermometer reaches 180 degrees in the thickest part.

When the chicken is halfway done, put the vegetables on the grill.

Sprinkle Italian seasoning over the chicken and vegetables to taste.

To serve, lay the grilled veggies on a plate, place the chicken breast on the grilled vegetables, and spoon the walnut sauce over the chicken and vegetables.

Serves 4.

Marinated Chicken

This meal has a bright, fresh taste from the combination of lemon and rosemary. Make extra to use in salads and sandwiches.

- 1/2 cup olive oil
- 2 tablespoon fresh rosemary
- 1 teaspoon minced garlic
- Juice and zest of 1 lemon
- 1/4 cup freshly chopped flat-leaf parsley
- Sea salt and freshly ground pepper, to taste
- 4 boneless, skinless chicken breasts

Mix the marinade ingredients together in a plastic bag or bowl.

Place the chicken in the container and shake/stir so the marinade thoroughly coats the chicken.

Refrigerate up to 24 hours.

Heat a grill to medium heat and cook the chicken for 6–8 minutes a side. Turn only once during the cooking process.

Serve with Greek salad and brown rice.

Serves 4.

Nicoise Chicken

This dish, inspired by Nice on the French Riviera, makes an easy and elegant meal—simple enough for every day, yet special enough for company. Don't skip the fresh tarragon, which really gives this dish some flair.

- 1/4 cup olive oil
- 3 medium onions, coarsely chopped
- 3 cloves garlic, minced
- 4 pounds chicken breast from 1 cut-up chicken
- 5 Roma tomatoes, peeled and chopped
- 1/2 cup white wine
- 1 (14 1/2-ounce) can chicken broth
- 1/2 cup black Nicoise olives
- Juice of 1 lemon
- 1/4 cup flat-leaf parsley, chopped
- 1 tablespoon fresh tarragon leaves, chopped
- Sea salt and freshly ground pepper, to taste

Heat the olive oil in a deep saucepan or stew pot over medium heat. Cook the onions and garlic 5 minutes, or until tender and translucent.

Add the chicken and cook an additional 5 minutes to brown slightly.

Add the tomatoes, white wine, and chicken broth, cover, and simmer 30–45 minutes on medium-low heat, or until the chicken is tender and the sauce is thickened slightly.

Remove the lid and add the olives and lemon juice.

Cook an additional 10–15 minutes to thicken the sauce further.

Stir in the parsley and tarragon, and salt and pepper to taste. Serve immediately.

Serves 6.

Rosemary Chicken

Quick and easy to make, this chicken dish can be served hot or cold. Try it chilled and sliced with a salad for lunch.

- Canola oil spray
- 1 (12-ounce) skinless chicken breast
- Freshly ground black pepper
- 4 medium tomatoes
- 1 tablespoon red wine vinegar
- 2 large sprigs fresh rosemary
- 1/2 cup dry white wine

Preheat the oven to 375 degrees.

Lightly coat an 8-inch glass baking dish with canola oil spray.

Arrange the chicken in the dish and dust generously with freshly ground black pepper.

Cut the tomatoes into quarters and arrange them around the chicken.

Sprinkle the vinegar over the tomatoes, then tuck the rosemary in next to the chicken.

Pour the wine into the dish, cover tightly with foil, and bake for 35 minutes.

Slice the chicken breast into bite-size pieces, toss with the rest of the ingredients, and serve.

Serves 2.

Turkey Fajitas

If you thought fajitas were no longer part of your menu plan, think again! Turkey replaces the beef, and Greek yogurt stands in for the sour cream.

- 1/2 pound fresh turkey breast
- 1/2 sweet red pepper, sliced
- 1/2 green pepper, diced
- 1 onion, sliced and divided
- 1 jalapeño pepper, seeded and chopped
- 20 green olives sliced
- 1 tablespoon olive oil
- 2 tablespoons prepared salsa, plus more for topping
- 2 whole-grain tortillas
- Chopped lettuce
- Greek yogurt
- Slice turkey into strips.

Heat oil in frying pan and add half the onion, the green and red pepper, and the jalapeño. Sauté for 5 minutes and add turkey.

Brown meat on all sides and add salsa.

Simmer for 20 minutes or until done.

Wrap tortillas in damp paper towels and microwave for 15–30 seconds.

Spoon turkey and vegetables onto tortillas, add remaining raw onion, chopped lettuce, Greek yogurt, and additional salsa as desired.

Serves 2.

White Chili

This mild chicken chili is perfect for potlucks and parties. Use any kind of white beans you like, such as great northern or cannellini beans. Top each serving with chopped fresh cilantro and green onions.

- 1 tablespoon olive oil
- 1 pound boneless, skinless chicken breasts or thighs, cut into 1-inch cubes
- 1 onion, chopped
- 2 (15 1/2-ounce) cans white beans, rinsed and drained
- 1 (14 1/2-ounce) can chicken broth
- 2 (4-ounce) cans green chilies, chopped
- 2 cloves garlic, minced
- 1/2 teaspoon sea salt
- 1 teaspoon ground cumin
- 1 teaspoon dried oregano
- Sea salt and freshly ground pepper, to taste

In a large Dutch oven, sauté the chicken and onion in olive oil for 5 minutes over medium-high heat.

Add the beans, broth, green chilies, garlic, salt, and spices. Bring to a boil, then lower the heat and simmer for 20 minutes.

Remove from heat and season with sea salt and freshly ground pepper to taste.

Serves 4.

FISH

Almond-Encrusted Salmon

Crushed almonds give this salmon a sweet and savory crunch. Salmon and almonds are both a good source of healthy fats. Make enough to use the leftovers in a green salad.

- 1/4 cup olive oil
- 1 tablespoon honey
- 1/2 cup finely chopped almonds, lightly toasted
- 1/2 teaspoon dried thyme
- Sea salt and freshly ground pepper, to taste
- 4 salmon steaks

Preheat the oven to 350 degrees.

Combine the olive oil with the honey. (Soften the honey in the microwave for 15 seconds, if necessary, for easier blending.)

In a shallow dish, combine the almonds, thyme, sea salt, and freshly ground pepper.

Coat the salmon steaks with the olive oil mixture, then the almond mixture.

Place on a baking sheet brushed with olive oil and bake 8–12 minutes, or until the almonds are lightly browned and the salmon is firm.

Serves 4.

Avocado Halibut

This fish dish has a bit of a kick, so beware of the heat. Serve with sliced fresh tomatoes and a green salad.

- Canola oil spray
- 2 (6-ounce) halibut fillets
- 2 ripe avocados, peeled and pitted
- 1/2 cup mild green salsa
- 1/2 cup nonfat Greek yogurt
- 1 fresh jalapeño, seeded and diced

Preheat the broiler.

Lightly coat a broiler pan with canola oil spray.

Mash the avocados and mix in the salsa, yogurt, and jalapeño.

Warm this mixture in a nonstick saucepan over low heat.

Place the halibut fillets on the broiler pan and broil for 5 minutes, then turn them over and broil another 4 minutes.

Serve the halibut with the warmed guacamole sauce on top.

Serves 2.

Baked Salmon with Capers and Olives

This fresh-tasting salmon dish is inspired by the cuisine of Greece and Italy, sans bread crumbs.

- 1 tablespoon olive oil
- 4 salmon steaks
- Sea salt and freshly ground pepper, to taste
- 2 Roma tomatoes, chopped
- 1/4 cup chopped, pitted green olives
- 1 clove garlic, minced
- Juice of 1/2 lemon
- 1 teaspoon capers, rinsed and drained
- 1/2 teaspoon sugar

Preheat the oven to 375 degrees.

Brush a baking dish with olive oil. Place the salmon fillets in the dish.

Season with sea salt and freshly ground pepper.

In a large bowl, combine all the remaining ingredients.

Top the salmon fillets with the tomato mixture.

Drizzle with olive oil and bake for 15 minutes, or until medium rare.

Serves 4.

Balsamic-Glazed Black-Pepper Salmon

Salmon is a rich and fatty fish that is very healthy. Choose wild Pacific salmon whenever possible. This dish pairs well with a light Pinot Noir.

- 1/2 cup balsamic vinegar
- 1 tablespoon honey
- 4 (8-ounce) salmon fillets
- Sea salt and freshly ground pepper, to taste
- 1 tablespoon olive oil

Heat a cast-iron skillet over medium-high heat.

Mix the balsamic vinegar and honey in a small bowl.

Season the salmon fillets with the sea salt and freshly ground pepper; brush with the honey-balsamic glaze.

Add olive oil to the skillet and sear the salmon fillets, cooking for 3–4 minutes on each side until lightly browned and medium rare in the center.

Let sit for 5 minutes before serving.

Serves 4.

Burgundy Salmon

Red wine is usually associated with beef, but here it complements rich salmon. Wild salmon is a healthier choice for you and the environment than farmed Atlantic salmon. Serve this dish with plenty of fresh green vegetables.

- 4 salmon steaks
- Sea salt and freshly ground pepper, to taste
- 1 tablespoon olive oil
- 1 shallot, minced
- 2 cups high-quality burgundy wine
- 1/2 cup beef stock
- 2 tablespoons tomato paste
- 1 teaspoon fresh thyme, chopped

Preheat the oven to 350 degrees.

Season the salmon steaks with sea salt and freshly ground pepper. Wrap the salmon steaks in aluminum foil and bake for 10–13 minutes.

Heat the olive oil in a deep skillet on medium heat. Add the shallot and cook for 3 minutes, or until tender.

Add the wine, beef stock, and tomato paste, and simmer for 10 minutes, or until sauce thickens and reduces by a third.

Place the fish on a serving platter and spoon the sauce over it.

Sprinkle the fish with the fresh thyme and serve.

Serves 4.

Grilled Bluefish

The citrus in this dish lends it a sunny flavor. If you can find small, whole bluefish, clean and grill them whole. Otherwise, fillets work fine. Bluefish is a good source of niacin, phosphorus, selenium, vitamin B6, and vitamin B12.

- 1 cup olive oil
- 1/2 cup white wine
- 1/4 cup fresh basil leaves, chopped
- Juice and zest of 2 lemons or oranges
- 2–3 garlic cloves, minced
- 1 teaspoon ground cumin
- 1 teaspoon thyme
- 2 pinches of cayenne pepper
- 4 bluefish or fish fillets
- Sea salt and freshly ground pepper, to taste

Combine all the ingredients except the fish in a plastic bag or shallow bowl.

Divide marinade in half, reserving half in the refrigerator and placing the fish in the other half of the marinade.

Refrigerate for at least 1 hour.

Heat the grill to medium-high heat. Brush the grates with olive oil.

Grill the fish for 6–8 minutes, turning halfway through the cooking time.

Warm the reserved marinade and serve with the fish. Season with salt and pepper to taste.

Serves 4.

Halibut with Roasted Vegetables

Halibut is a firm, mild fish that pairs well with a variety of seasonings and vegetables. Here, it's combined with tomatoes and zucchinis. Feel free to improvise with what's available in your garden or farmers' market.

- 1/2 cup olive oil
- 1/4 cup small white mushrooms, coarsely chopped
- 2 small tomatoes, coarsely chopped
- 1 small white onion, chopped
- 2 zucchinis, chopped
- 2 cloves garlic, minced
- 1 teaspoon Herbs de Provence
- Sea salt and freshly ground pepper, to taste
- 1 1/2 pounds halibut steak, cut into 6 pieces
- 3 tablespoons fresh tarragon, chopped finely
- Juice of 1 lemon

Preheat the oven to 350 degrees.

Toss the mushrooms, vegetables, and herbs on a large baking sheet with the olive oil and season with sea salt and freshly ground pepper.

Roast for 15–20 minutes, or until soft and slightly browned. Do not burn.

Place the halibut steaks on another baking sheet and season with the tarragon, sea salt, freshly ground pepper, and lemon juice.

Roast for 10–13 minutes.

Top the halibut steaks with the roasted vegetables.

Serves 6.

Herb-Marinated Flounder

Although dried herbs work in many recipes, fresh herbs are much tastier. Fresh herbs are also a better source of antioxidants than dry herbs. Most herbs grow easily in a pot on your back step, or even a sunny windowsill in your kitchen.

- 1/2 cup lightly packed flat-leaf parsley
- 1/4 cup olive oil
- 4 garlic cloves, peeled and halved
- 2 tablespoons fresh rosemary
- 2 tablespoons fresh thyme leaves
- 2 tablespoons fresh sage
- 2 tablespoons lemon zest
- Sea salt and freshly ground pepper, to taste
- 4 flounder fillets

Preheat the oven to 350 degrees.

Place all the ingredients except the fish in a food processor. Blend to form a thick paste.

Place the fillets on a baking sheet and brush paste on them. Refrigerate for at least 1 hour.

Bake for 8–10 minutes, or until the flounder is slightly firm and opaque.

Serves 4.

Poached Cod

Poaching is an ideal method for cooking soft fish, such as cod. Although this recipe calls for cod, substitute any white fish.

- 1 tablespoon olive oil
- 1/2 cup onion, thinly sliced
- 1 cup fennel, thinly sliced
- 1 tablespoon garlic, minced
- 1 (15-ounce) can diced tomatoes
- 2 cups chicken broth
- 1/2 cup white wine
- Juice and zest of 1 orange
- 1 pinch red pepper flakes
- 1 bay leaf
- 1 pound cod

Heat the olive oil in a large skillet. Add the onion and fennel, and cook 10 minutes, or until translucent and soft.

Add the garlic and cook 1 minute.

Add the tomatoes, chicken broth, wine, orange juice and zest, red pepper flakes, and bay leaf, and simmer for 5 minutes to meld the flavors.

Carefully add the fish in a single layer.

Cover and simmer 6–7 minutes.

Transfer fish to a serving dish and ladle the remaining sauce over the fish.

Serves 4.

Quick Fish Florentine

*Spinach is a classic accompaniment to fish. This quick and easy recipe has
no flour or breadcrumbs. Serve with rice.*

- 1 cup spinach, cooked
- 2 (6-ounce) flounder fillets, fresh or frozen and defrosted
- 2 tablespoons olive oil
- Sea salt and freshly ground pepper, to taste
- 1 teaspoon lemon juice
- 1 teaspoon lemon zest

Make two beds of spinach on a microwave-safe baking dish.

Coat fish with olive oil on both sides and season with sea salt and freshly
ground pepper.

Place fish on top of the spinach and microwave on high for 3–5 minutes,
until fish is opaque and flakes easily.

Drizzle the fish with lemon juice and sprinkle with zest before serving.

Serves 2.

Roasted Sea Bass

Roasting is an easy and forgiving way to prepare almost any fish. Use it to cook whole fish, fish fillets, or even fish chunks, and simply adjust the cooking time based on the fish's size. Enjoy this dish with sautéed greens.

- 1/4 cup olive oil
- Whole sea bass or fillets
- Sea salt and freshly ground pepper, to taste
- 1/4 cup dry white wine
- 3 teaspoons fresh dill
- 2 teaspoons fresh thyme
- 1 garlic clove, minced

Preheat the oven to 425 degrees.

Brush the bottom of a roasting pan with olive oil. Place the fish in the pan and brush the fish with oil.

Season fish with sea salt and freshly ground pepper.

Combine the remaining ingredients and pour over the fish.

Bake for 10–15 minutes, depending on the size of the fish.

Sea bass is done when the flesh is firm and opaque.

Serves 6.

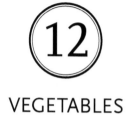

VEGETABLES

Braised Eggplant and Tomatoes

This thick vegetarian ragù is delicious enough to eat over a grain. Getting your daily allowance of vegetables is easy with a dish like this.

- 1 large eggplant, peeled and diced
- Pinch of sea salt
- 1 (15-ounce) can chopped tomatoes and juices
- 1 cup chicken broth
- 2 smashed garlic cloves
- 1 tablespoon Italian seasoning
- Sea salt and freshly ground pepper, to taste
- 1 bay leaf

Cut the eggplant into 1/2-inch slices and salt both sides to remove bitter juices. Let the eggplant sit for 20 minutes before rinsing and patting dry.

Cube eggplant.

Put eggplant, tomatoes, chicken broth, garlic, seasonings, and bay leaf in a large saucepot.

Bring to a boil and reduce heat to simmer.

Cover and simmer for about 30–40 minutes, until eggplant is tender.

Remove garlic cloves and bay leaf. Salt and pepper to taste, and serve.

Serves 4.

Caramelized Root Vegetables

Cooking the vegetables in this recipe slowly will allow them to develop color and sweetness without burning. Don't skip the seasonings—spices have nutrients and antioxidant power.

- 2 medium carrots, cut into chunks
- 2 medium red and gold beets, cut into chunks
- 2 turnips, peeled and cut into chunks
- 2 tablespoons olive oil
- 1 teaspoon cumin
- 1 teaspoon sweet paprika
- Sea salt and freshly ground pepper, to taste
- Juice of 1 lemon
- 1 small bunch parsley, chopped

Preheat oven to 400 degrees.

Toss the vegetables with the olive oil and seasonings. Season with sea salt and freshly ground pepper.

Lay in a single layer on a sheet pan, cover with lemon juice, and roast for 30–40 minutes, until veggies are slightly browned and crisp.

Serve warm, topped with the chopped parsley.

Serves 6.

Grilled Vegetables

Less fat doesn't have to mean less flavor. Here, balsamic vinegar adds pizzazz to a variety of grilled vegetables. Feel free to substitute vegetables.

- 4 carrots, peeled and cut in half
- 2 onions, quartered
- 1 zucchini, cut into 1/2-inch rounds
- 1 red bell pepper, seeded and cut into cubes
- 1/4 cup olive oil
- Sea salt and freshly ground pepper, to taste
- Balsamic vinegar

Heat the grill to medium-high heat.

Brush the vegetables lightly with olive oil and season with sea salt and freshly ground pepper.

Place the carrots and onions on the grill first because they take the longest.

Cook the vegetables for 3–4 minutes on each side.

Transfer to a serving dish and drizzle with olive oil and balsamic vinegar.

Serves 4.

Mushroom-Stuffed Zucchini

Fresh zucchinis with mushrooms seasoned with garlic, olive oil, parsley, and herbs and spices hardly seems like diet food. These mushroom-stuffed zucchini boats make an easy and impressive dish that is low in calories but still filling. Serve with a piece of fish, or serve alone for a light lunch.

- 2 tablespoons olive oil
- 2 cups button mushrooms, finely chopped
- 2 cloves garlic, finely chopped
- 2 tablespoons chicken broth
- 1 tablespoon fresh parsley, finely chopped
- 1 tablespoon Italian seasoning
- Sea salt and freshly ground pepper, to taste
- 2 medium zucchinis, cut in half lengthwise

Preheat your oven to 350 degrees.

Heat a large skillet over medium heat and add the olive oil. Add the mushrooms and cook until tender, about 4 minutes.

Add the garlic and cook for 2 more minutes.

Add the chicken broth and cook another 3–4 minutes

Add the parsley and Italian seasoning, and season with sea salt and freshly ground pepper.

Stir and remove from heat.

Scoop out the insides of the halved zucchinis and stuff the mushroom mixture into the zucchinis.

Put them in a casserole dish and drizzle a tablespoon of water or broth in the bottom.

Cover with foil and bake for 30–40 minutes, until zucchinis are tender.

Serve immediately.

Serves 2.

Roasted Beets with Oranges and Onions

When combined with the oranges in this dish, roasted beets become extra sweet and special. Beets are a great source of phytonutrients, so finding more ways to enjoy them will also boost your health.

- 4 medium beets, trimmed and scrubbed
- Juice and zest of 2 oranges
- 1 red onion, thinly sliced
- 2 tablespoons olive oil
- 1 tablespoon red wine vinegar
- Juice of 1 lemon
- Sea salt and freshly ground pepper, to taste

Preheat oven to 400 degrees.

Wrap the beets in a foil pack and close tightly. Place them on a baking sheet and roast 40 minutes, until tender enough to be pierced easily with a knife.

Cool until easy to handle.

Combine the beets with the orange juice and zest, red onion, olive oil, vinegar, and lemon juice.

Season with sea salt and freshly ground pepper to taste and toss lightly.

Allow to sit for about 15 minutes for the flavors to meld before serving.

Serves 6.

Roasted Vegetable Pizza

This vegetable pizza will satisfy the craving for a food most everyone loves. Experiment with different combinations of roasted vegetables, and if you can't find a whole-grain pizza crust, consider this your treat for the week.

- 1 bunch asparagus, washed and trimmed, cut into 3-inch pieces
- 1 red onion, sliced into half rounds
- 1 red pepper, cored and sliced
- 1 cup mushrooms, sliced
- 1 small eggplant, ends trimmed, cut into quarter rounds
- 2 tablespoons olive oil
- 1 whole-grain pizza crust
- 1/4 cup pizza sauce
- 1/2 cup low-fat mozzarella cheese, grated
- 1 teaspoon Italian herb blend

Preheat oven to 400 degrees.

Arrange vegetables in 1 or 2 roasting pans, to accommodate a single layer. Drizzle with olive oil and toss until evenly coated.

Arrange in single layer and transfer to the oven.

Roast for 15–20 minutes or until tender. Remove from oven.

Spread sauce over the crust in a thin layer.

Arrange vegetables and sprinkle evenly with mozzarella and herbs. (Do not overload the pizza. There will be leftover vegetables and sauce. They can be stored in the refrigerator and used later on sandwiches, salads, or pasta.)

Bake pizza for 5–10 minutes, until cheese is melted and crust is crisp.

Serves 4.

Rosemary-Roasted Acorn Squash

When roasted at high heat, the skin of acorn squash becomes soft, tender, and edible. Rosemary is thought to stimulate the immune system, increase circulation, and improve digestion.

- 1 acorn squash
- 2 tablespoons honey
- 2 tablespoons rosemary, finely chopped
- 2 tablespoons olive oil
- Sea salt, to taste

Preheat oven to 400 degrees.

Cut your squash in half and clean out the seeds. Slice each half into 4 wedges.

Mix honey, rosemary, and olive oil.

Lay squash on baking sheet and sprinkle each slice with a bit of the mixture and a touch of sea salt.

Turn over and sprinkle other side.

Bake for approximately 30 minutes, or until squash is tender and slightly caramelized. Turn each slice over halfway through.

Serve immediately.

Serves 4.

Sautéed Crunchy Greens

If you're looking for a super-low-calorie dish, you can't go wrong with greens. There is no other food that is as low calorie and nutrient dense, so enjoy! Sunflower seeds are high in vitamin E, vitamin B1, manganese, copper, tryptophan, magnesium, selenium, and more.

- 3 tablespoons olive oil
- 2 cloves garlic, minced
- 2 large bunches Swiss chard or kale, sliced stems removed
- Juice of 1/2 lemon
- Sea salt and freshly ground pepper, to taste
- 3 tablespoons sunflower seeds

In a large skillet, heat the olive oil and add the garlic on medium heat. Sauté for about 1 minute and add the Swiss chard.

Cook until wilted, about 2 more minutes.

Add the lemon juice, sea salt, and freshly ground pepper to taste, then add sunflower seeds.

Serve and enjoy!

Serves 4.

Sautéed Mustard Greens and Red Peppers

Add a pinch of red chili flakes if you want a bit more spice in this scrumptious veggie delight.

- 1 tablespoon olive oil
- 1/2 red bell pepper, diced
- 2 cloves garlic, minced
- 1 bunch mustard greens
- Sea salt and freshly ground pepper, to taste
- 1 teaspoon white wine vinegar

Heat olive oil in a large saucepan over medium heat. Add bell pepper and garlic and sauté for 1 minute, stirring often.

Add greens to pan and immediately cover to begin steaming. Set a timer for 2 minutes.

After 1 minute, lift lid and stir greens well, then immediately put lid back on for remaining minute. Remove the lid, season with sea salt and freshly ground pepper, sprinkle with vinegar, and serve.

Serves 4.

Stuffed Cucumbers

Cucumbers contain a lot of water but also have antioxidant and anti-inflammatory properties. This juicy summer treat makes a great side dish or snack.

- 1 English cucumber
- 1 tomato, diced
- 1 avocado, diced
- Dash of lime juice
- Sea salt and freshly ground pepper, to taste

Small bunch cilantro, chopped

Cut the cucumber in half lengthwise and scoop out the flesh and seeds into a small bowl.

Without mashing too much, gently combine the cucumber flesh and seeds with the tomato, avocado, and lime juice.

Season with sea salt and freshly ground pepper to taste.

Put mixture back into cucumber halves and cut each piece in half.

Garnish with the cilantro and serve.

Serves 2.

Swiss Chard with White Beans and Bell Peppers

Beans are cheap, nutritional powerhouses that fill you up. Use a red bell pepper whenever possible in recipes that call for bell peppers: they are riper and have more nutrients.

- 2 tablespoons olive oil
- 1 medium onion, chopped
- 1 bell pepper, diced
- 2 cloves garlic, minced
- 1 large bunch of Swish chard, tough stems removed, cut into bite-size pieces
- 2 cups white beans, cooked
- Sea salt and freshly ground pepper, to taste

Heat the oil in a large skillet over medium-high heat. Add the onion and pepper and cook for 5 minutes until soft.

Add the garlic, stir, and add the Swiss chard. Cook for 10 minutes until greens are tender.

Add the beans, stir until heated through, and season with sea salt and freshly ground pepper.

Serve immediately.

Serves 4.

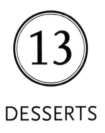

DESSERTS

Berry Parfait

Greek yogurt and berries is a combination you can enjoy without guilt! Use one type of berry or a combination. Enjoy this as a breakfast, snack, or dessert.

- 1/2 cup fresh berries, such as blueberries, raspberries, or blackberries

- 1 cup vanilla-flavored Greek yogurt
- 1/4 cup Crunchy Granola (see page 34)

Put half the berries in a parfait glass and top with the yogurt.

Top with the rest of the berries and the granola.

Serve immediately.

Serves 1.

Cocoa and Coconut Banana Slices

Frozen bananas have a creamy consistency that mimics ice cream. Bananas are a good source of dietary fiber, vitamin C, potassium, and manganese. This dessert also makes a great snack for adults or kids.

- 1 banana, sliced
- 2 tablespoons unsweetened, shredded coconut
- 1 tablespoon unsweetened cocoa powder
- 1 teaspoon honey

Lay the banana slices on a parchment-lined baking sheet in a single layer.

Put in the freezer for about 10 minutes, until firm but not frozen solid.

Mix the coconut with the cocoa powder in a small bowl.

Roll the banana slices in honey, followed by the coconut mixture.

You can either eat immediately or put back in the freezer for a frozen sweet treat.

Serves 1.

Cucumber Lime Popsicles

These popsicles are a delicious and refreshing way to consume antioxidants. Adults and kids alike love these easy-to-make summer treats.

- 2 cups cold water
- 1 cucumber, peeled
- 1/4 cup honey
- Juice of 1 lime

In a blender, puree the water, cucumbers, honey, and lime juice.

Pour into popsicle molds, freeze, and enjoy on a hot summer day!

Serves 4–6.

Frozen Raspberry Delight

You can make a sorbet-style treat with frozen fruit. This dessert will help you meet your daily requirement for fruit. Swap the peach or mango for a banana if you prefer.

• 3 cups frozen raspberries	• 1 mango, peeled and pitted
• 1 peach, peeled and pitted	• 1 teaspoon honey

Add all ingredients to a blender and puree, only adding enough water to keep the mixture moving and your blender from overworking itself.

Freeze for 10 minutes to firm up if desired.

Serves 2.

Overnight Jam

Use this jam with the Thumbprint Cookies in this section or with a piece of whole-grain bread.

- 1/4 cup dried apricots
- 1/4 cup dried cherries
- 1/2 cup dried apples
- Pinch of sea salt

Roughly chop all fruits and put in bowl with sea salt and cover with water.

Cover bowl and refrigerate for 12 hours or overnight until fruit is plump. Drain excess water and place in food processor or blender.

Blend until you have a thick, chunky jam.

Store tightly sealed in refrigerator for up to 2 weeks.

Yields 1 cup.

Red Wine Poached Pears

Pears are a low-calorie fruit and a good source of fiber. These make a delicious dessert but are also lovely alongside rich dishes as well.

- 2 cups red wine, such as merlot or zinfandel, more if necessary
- 2 firm pears, peeled
- 2–3 cardamom pods, split
- 1 cinnamon stick
- 2 peppercorns
- 1 bay leaf

Put all ingredients in a large pot and bring to a boil.

Make sure the pears are submerged in the wine.

Reduce heat and simmer for 15–20 minutes, until the pears are tender when poked with a fork.

Remove the pears from the wine and allow to cool.

Bring the wine to a boil and cook until it reduces to a syrup.

Strain and drizzle the pears with the warmed syrup before serving.

Serves 2.

Thumbprint Cookies

These wheat-free cookies will rock your world, but they won't mess with your diet.

- 1 cup raw almonds
- 1 cup rolled oats
- 1 cup organic spelt flour
- 1/2 teaspoon cinnamon
- 1/2 teaspoon powdered ginger
- 1/8 teaspoon nutmeg
- 1/4 teaspoon sea salt
- 1/2 cup canola oil
- 1/2 cup honey
- 1 teaspoon vanilla extract
- Overnight Jam (see page 138) for filling

Preheat oven to 350 degrees, and line a cookie pan with parchment paper.

Use a food processor with metal blade to grind almonds into coarse flour, about 2 minutes.

Add oats, flour, cinnamon, ginger, nutmeg, and sea salt, and process for 1 more minute.

Add oil, honey, and vanilla extract, and continue to process until dough forms a ball.

Wrap dough in plastic wrap and set aside for 15 minutes at room temperature.

Using a tablespoon of dough, form balls and place on cookie sheet. Make a thumbprint in each cookie and fill with Overnight Jam.

Bake about 15 minutes, until cookie bottoms are browned.

Serves 6.

Tropical Sorbet

Fresh fruit is the basis for this very refreshing sorbet. It can also be served as a palate cleanser between courses. Substitute tangerine juice for the orange juice, for a more exotic flavor.

- 2 cups fresh pineapple, cut into 2-inch pieces
- 2 cups fresh mango, sliced
- 2 tablespoons honey
- 2 tablespoons freshly squeezed orange juice

Line a jelly roll pan with plastic wrap.

Arrange fruit in 1 layer.

Cover and seal with more plastic wrap and freeze overnight.

Transfer frozen fruit to the food processor and pulse until finely chopped.

Add honey and orange juice and process for 30 seconds.

Taste and add more honey if necessary. Blend for 5 minutes or until very smooth, scraping down the sides a few times.

Spoon into a tightly covered container and return to freezer.

Transfer to the refrigerator for 20 minutes before scooping and serving.

Serves 4.

Made in the USA
Middletown, DE
27 December 2016